The
Clothesline
Diet

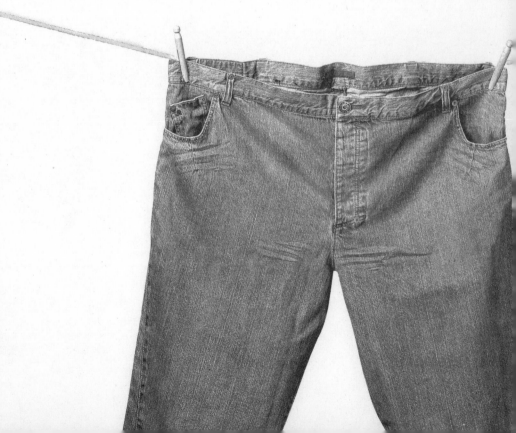

The Clothesline Diet

The Incredible Story of
How One Woman
Went from **Flab to Fab**
and How You Can, Too!

KAREN GATT
with SUE SMETHURST

HARLEQUIN™
THE CLOTHESLINE DIET

ISBN-13: 978-0-373-89219-8

The ideas, procedures and suggestions contained in this book are not intended as a substitute for consulting with your physician. All matters regarding your health require medical supervision.

Library of Congress
Cataloging-in-Publication Data
Gatt, Karen
The Clothesline Diet
The Incredible Story of How One Woman
Went from Flab to Fab and How You Can, Too!
Karen Gatt with Sue Smethurst
p. cm.
Includes index.
ISBN 978-0-373-89219-8 (pbk.)
1. Diet. I. Gatt Karen II. Title.
TT670.C37 2009
646.4'204--dc22
2008051431

Lina's after photo (Chapter 5) by David Mason

www.eHarlequin.com

Printed in U.S.A.

It only takes

one step

to change

your life.

CONTENTS

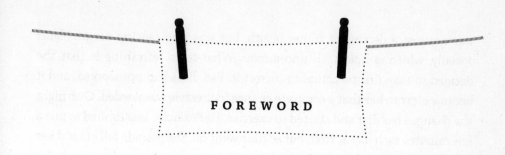

A Doctor's View

OBESITY HAS BECOME A PROBLEM OF EPIDEMIC PROPORTIONS IN the United States and is becoming a problem of similar proportions in other countries such as Australia where a Western diet is prevalent. Due to the spreading of the Western diet, countries that have traditionally eaten Eastern diets low in fat and salt are now experiencing similar obesity trends, particularly in China, where childhood obesity is becoming a major health concern.

In my practice I have several patients who are morbidly obese, weighing upward of 300 pounds or more. When interviewing those patients, I found several common lifestyle features: First, they consume enormous amounts of calories on a daily basis. Second, they have a sedentary lifestyle.

When I first heard about Karen Gatt's book, I read it with great interest and found her experiences to be typical of the experiences of many of my patients. Many, like Karen, were overweight as children. As they grew into adulthood, they became more sedentary and continued their dietary indiscretions, eating highly processed high-fat foods as well as foods with high sugar content and without the nutritious benefits of the fruits, vegetables, grains and poultry that are the mainstays of the western diet.

Karen found herself in an intolerable situation. She realized her weight was not just a detriment to her health, but was also causing her problems socially, which is not at all uncommon. What is so refreshing is that she decided to take drastic action to correct it. Fad diets had not worked, and it became clear to her that a complete change in lifestyle was needed. Overnight she changed her diet and started to exercise. Her exercise was limited to just a few minutes each day at first, but as time went on, the pounds fell off and her endurance improved, as did her self-esteem.

Within thirteen months she shed 150 pounds, a phenomenal achievement, but it is especially significant because she represents hope. To those who've lost hope and think they cannot shed the weight they've carried around all these years, or will never wear a "normal-sized" dress or pair of pants, Karen's experience represents a light in the darkness of despair.

Her book, *The Clothesline Diet,* is the first of several she has written about her experience. Here in California, I invited Karen to speak to a group of my patients. She gave each and every one of them a spark of hope; if she could do it, so could they. As Karen makes clear, it is simply a matter of changing one's lifestyle.

It is my fervent hope that her enthusiasm and sincerity to help those who are struggling with their weight will spread to this continent someday. We as physicians can tell our patients to lose weight. However it takes effort and a strong will as well as strong family and peer support to do it. This is where Karen comes in. We in America can certainly use someone with her common sense and determination.

Albert Bodt, M.D.
Division of Nephrology
Department of Internal Medicine,
Kaiser Permanente Medical Offices
Lancaster, California

Awakening the New Me

OH MY GOD. IT'S ALMOST IMPOSSIBLE TO BEGIN TO TELL YOU how much my life has changed over the past eight years. To go from being a mother of two toddlers who was so obese I could barely squeeze through my front door to "Australia's favorite diet mum," as the press have dubbed me, with people all around the world following *my* weight-loss plan is...unbelievable! I still pinch myself every day.

When I first started on my weight-loss journey, walking around the clothesline in my backyard, I weighed almost 300 pounds. I lost 150 pounds—that's actually a whole person—on my own by devising a simple diet plan and walking tiny laps of the clothesline in my backyard. No pills, no potions, no gimmicks, no prepackaged meals, no points to count. Trust me, I'd tried all of the fad diets so many times I'd lost count, and none of them worked for me. But this diet did. Why? I think it's because it's a real down under diet—it's simple and straightforward with no bulldust. I'm not a doctor or a dietician, I'm just a mum who spent most of her life struggling to get off the diet roller coaster. I finally did it by following a simple diet I created myself, literally in my own backyard. I'm

I'm not a doctor or a dietician, I'm just a mum who spent most of my life struggling to get off the diet roller coaster.

not an educated person, but I made my dream come true—and if I can do it, anyone can.

In 1999 I hit rock bottom. I weighed nearly 300 pounds and my self-esteem was so low I often wondered if life was worth living. I was disgusted with myself.

Normal day-to-day behavior that thin people take for granted—like talking to friends and going shopping or, for that matter, any activity that made me step outside my home—became a terrifying ordeal. I had quite literally eaten my life away. I could barely walk to the mailbox, let alone play with my two toddler sons or try on a pair of jeans at the local mall. I avoided playing with my kids because I simply couldn't keep up with them; I'd have to lie down and have a rest afterward. My poor knees felt like they were crumbling under the weight of my enormous body. There were days when I would do a load of laundry and actually feel as if I were having a heart attack from lifting the clothes into the washing machine—and I was only twenty-six years old!

I made my dream come true—and if I can do it, anyone can.

My house had become a physical and mental fortress. It was the only place where I felt safe, away from the stares, whispers, taunts and sheer disgust that overwhelmed me every time I stepped outside the door. I hated having to get ready to go out somewhere—my home offered me protection, and the mere thought of having to face the world sparked an unbearable anxiety for me. What was the point of making an effort to do my hair, or put on some makeup when, in my eyes, I was still the same ugly, overweight Karen no matter what I was wearing.

I hated how I looked and who I had become.

Most women, as they go to leave the house, will have one last look in the mirror to make sure their hair is in place and their lipstick is right. I always had one last look in the mirror, too. But not to admire myself.

I would turn to the mirror and spit at myself in sheer disgust because I hated how I looked and who I had become. I would stand there, staring at myself until the very last dribble of saliva had run down over the reflection of my face while tears rolled down my cheeks. I hated myself so much, and I loathed the way I looked and felt. I had reached the lowest point of my life, and I was drained of all self-esteem. This was my routine every time I left the house.

My wardrobe was a constant source of depression. Sliding back the closet doors to the racks of "fat" clothes would remind me of the life I didn't have and, worse, the life I did. All of the clothes were the same—straight fitting, size 24 to 26, an array of bright colors and patterns supposedly designed to disguise my weight. The theory was that the bigger the shirts, the more they would hide the rolls of fat bulging beneath, but in reality there were few clothes that could hide my rippling roly-poly shape.

My ultimate nightmare was going out with my husband, Jason, like a normal married couple. Hours before we were due to leave the house, I would begin to worry about what I was going to wear. Popping something on a few minutes before we were due to walk out the door, like slim women can do, just wasn't an option. I tried on each piece of clothing that I peeled off the hanger over and over again, until eventually I'd tortured myself so much and was so frustrated that I would lie on the bed and cry my eyes out. Nothing looked right, or felt right, and in the end I would be so angry with myself for being overweight that I would grab the first thing I saw and put it on, even though I'd tried it on four or five times already.

The tears, the hatred and the anguish didn't happen once in a while—this was how I lived all the time, every day.

The tears, the hatred and the anguish didn't happen once in a while—this was how I lived all the time, every day. This was what my life had become, and all because of my weight.

After the tears I would try to convince myself that I didn't care what people thought. They would like me for who I was, for my personality. But somewhere in my head, eating away at me constantly, was the truth—I did care what people thought.

The Courage to Change

All of this changed for me during a Mother's Day dinner-dance in May 1999. I remember it as if it were yesterday. I really didn't want to go, but Jason and my children, four-year-old Brendan and three-year-old Ryan, were so looking forward to it.

I dreaded walking into any room full of people and this night was no different. All the mums in the ballroom that night were so beautiful—except me. I felt so embarrassed about the way I looked and, as we walked into the hall to find our table, it felt like every pair of eyes in the room was staring right at me. Here I was wearing something that resembled a tent, plodding across the dance floor like a baby elephant, desperate to get to our table so I could sit down and hide myself. What I would have given for the ground to open up and swallow me right then and there.

Aside from the sheer embarrassment, I was disgusted with myself. Disgusted that I had gotten myself into this situation. Disgusted that I was so big, and angry that I had allowed myself to get this overweight. I couldn't believe how fat I had become and I had no one to blame but me—nobody else shoved food into my mouth, it was my own fault. Dropping my head as low as I could so as to avoid all of their faces, I sat straight down in my chair. I just wanted to die.

I couldn't believe how fat I had become and I had no one to blame but me.

This was supposed to be a night of celebration, so when the band struck up and they invited all of the mothers onto the dance floor with their partners, Jason grabbed my hand and said, "C'mon, Kaz, let's go." He was only trying to do the right thing, but I refused. It felt like every eye in the room was on me, the fat girl.

Jason could sense I was upset and kept pushing me to dance, thinking it would cheer me up. Feeling so guilty that I was spoiling his fun, I agreed to get up, and as the band began to play we took to the floor. We lasted half a song before I made the excuse that I needed to use the bathroom and fled from the crowd.

People probably weren't staring at all, but I felt like the whole world was watching, and I was desperately embarrassed. I just wanted to hide. I felt like I didn't fit in. I was so uncomfortable dancing in front of people that I had to get away. The restrooms were close to where we were dancing, so I didn't have to walk past too many people, and once inside, I could hide from prying eyes and my problems would disappear for a moment.

I closed the door of the cubicle and sat on the toilet seat for about fifteen minutes, praying to be taken home. I stayed there for what felt like forever.

The other women must have wondered what was going on. There was a huge line but I didn't care. I wasn't getting out for anyone. I buried my face in my hands and rocked backward and forward, blocking the world out of my mind to comfort myself before I finally built up enough courage to walk back out.

I didn't look at any of their faces—I just brushed past them all, went straight back to my chair and sat staring around the room at the other mothers. All the mothers that night looked so happy; they were smiling, laughing, having a great night out with their husbands and families. After all, isn't that how life is meant to be? They were the center of attention on Mother's Day. It was their night to celebrate, but I didn't feel much like celebrating with them.

From that precise moment I knew I had to change my life.

I spent a lot of that night just looking around the room at all the other women, staring and admiring the clothes they wore, how their hair was done so nicely and how beautiful they all looked. Most of them were older than me, and yet they were living the life I wanted to live. They looked the way I wanted to look. They smiled the way I wanted to smile.

And here I was, twenty-six years old with two beautiful children and a gorgeous husband, wearing a size 26: so fat that I struggled to walk, carrying the weight of the world on my shoulders.

As I looked at their faces, something inside of me clicked. From that precise moment I knew I had to change my life. I knew that I deserved to smile and laugh just like them. I wanted to look and feel gorgeous, no matter what I had on. I just wanted to be part of the real world and, most of all, I wanted to live a normal life. No more huffing and puffing and no more sadness—I wanted the life I'd never had.

My life was going to change—and it did.

People treated me very differently when I was obese; they'd look at me with pity or laugh at me. I was never treated as an equal and it destroyed me, slowly eating away at my confidence.

Jason and I barely spoke in the car going home that night—my mind was too busy dwelling on the changes I was going to make. So many things were going through my head.

We got into bed and Jason fell asleep straightaway, but not me. I lay there for hours wondering about the future I longed to have. There was something stirring deep down inside me—and it wasn't food! I knew that when I got out of bed the next morning, the steps I took would be the first toward a new me. My life was going to change—and it did.

The First Small Steps

I woke up at 7:00 a.m., got up and made myself a cup of coffee. The kids and Jason were still in bed asleep and the whole house was blissfully silent. I sat quietly at the kitchen table, sipping my coffee, going over and reinforcing my goals in my head.

Over breakfast I plucked up the courage to tell Jason about my dreams.

"This is the day I'm going to turn my life around," I told him, but he just looked at me and rolled his eyes and said, "Here we go again."

I don't blame him—boy, hadn't he heard it all before! His lack of faith was understandable because I had tried to lose weight so many times I'd lost count. I think there's barely a diet plan, weight-loss potion, lotion, pill or gimmick that I haven't tried. The soup diet, the water diet, the starvation diet! You name it, I've tried them all, and I couldn't count the number of diet pills I've taken. I hate to think now what all of that was doing to my body.

I had tried to lose weight so many times I'd lost count.

But it was at our kitchen table that morning where I started the journey that has changed my whole world and given me a second chance at life.

I knew this time that I really had to change; I had to lose weight. If I didn't I would die—I was dying on the inside anyway and I didn't think I could continue to face the world if this wasn't a success and I let everybody down yet again. I had to make it work.

In my heart I really knew I could change and I could make myself happy.

In my heart I really knew I could change and I could make myself happy. It was just a matter of making it happen. I was always smiling on the outside. I was happy-go-lucky, "bubbly" Karen. I was the extrovert, always the life of the party. Nobody could see how much I hated myself and how much I was hurting on the inside. But a few seconds away from people and I would be in tears, constantly.

It's amazing how much your mind controls you—until that morning I'd never really allowed myself to believe I *could* change my life. It was always in the back of my mind, but I would make excuses for myself: "You're so fat you don't deserve to be happy." And I would actually talk myself into believing that I should be unhappy because I had made myself fat.

When I started to believe in myself, it dawned on me that for the first time, it wasn't my head talking, but my heart. This was different from all the other attempts, because the need to get my life back came from somewhere deep inside. It wasn't a thought that my mind could just discard, it was a desperate shift within my soul. It was almost as if there was someone else inside me, telling me I could do this, making me listen and not accepting any of the excuses I had used before.

The feeling was so overwhelming that in some ways it felt like my own angel from God had come to rescue me.

Living with Obesity

When you're as obese as I was, your weight is on your mind all the time.

I used to stand outside shop windows in the mall and stare for what felt like forever at the beautiful clothes on display. I'd go inside and touch them and long to be able to wear them, but in my heart I knew that those jeans would barely stretch over one leg. Instead of doing what most people would think was the logical thing to do and resolving to lose the weight, the depression would send me on an eating binge. I'd head straight to the food court to devour everything in sight: pizzas, french fries, everything. And I'm not talking about one slice of pizza or a couple of fries, I'm talking about the whole lot in one sitting. Sometimes I'd have three or four pieces of pizza and I'd feel so guilty halfway through the second or third, I'd stop eating. But an hour or so later I'd go back and get another slice, then top it off with an ice cream. For a few minutes food seemed to take away all of the pain of being overweight, but soon I'd feel so disappointed in myself and so ashamed that I'd go home, lock myself in the bedroom and cry for hours.

For a few minutes food seemed to take away all of the pain of being overweight, but soon I'd feel so disappointed in myself that I'd cry for hours.

This kind of behavior wasn't just an "every now and then" thing. This was how I lived my life every single day. I longed to lose weight, but I told myself it was just a silly dream that I could never achieve.

Today my life has totally turned around—all because, finally, I believed in myself and listened to my heart.

Believing Is a Gift of Life

On the afternoon of New Year's Eve 2001 I went to my closet and pulled out the most beautiful black beaded dress. After one year of dieting, I was so confident. I felt beautiful and I was on top of the world. It was the first time I had happily worn a dress since my wedding in 1990. In the past dresses had always made me feel so fat. But this night was different.

Today, my life has totally turned around—all because, finally, I believed in myself.

We were going to a New Year's Eve dinner-dance and a few weeks before, I'd found this dress while I was out shopping. It was the first one I tried on and bingo! It was perfect. It was a bit of a splurge, but to me it was worth the money. After missing out on wearing dresses for so many years, I thought I deserved this one.

When the day came I started to get ready hours beforehand as usual—but this time I loved every second of it. I didn't want to waste a moment. When I walked out of the bedroom, Jason was sitting on the couch, wide-eyed and totally speechless. He finally managed to stutter, "You look absolutely gorgeous—I'm so proud of you...it's an honor to have you as my wife."

My boys, Brendan and Ryan, couldn't stop staring at me. Brendan said, "Mummy, you look so pretty," and Ryan told me I was beautiful. That was the most amazing feeling. I was overwhelmed and so happy. I'd lost nearly 150 pounds and I'd found my self-esteem and my confidence again.

That night, we walked into the party and I was *hoping* everybody was looking at me; I was so proud of myself and I felt like I was walking on air. There were seven hundred people in that room already seated, and some of them stared in disbelief. I didn't look down at the floor, I didn't hurry to sit down, I walked slowly, confidently, and I savored every second—I was making the most of each moment. The feeling was incredible, like nothing I'd ever felt before.

The band began to play and they invited everybody onto the dance floor. Jason and I looked at each other, nodded and made our way into the crowd. We danced and danced, song after song. I knew exactly how Cinderella felt when she was dancing at the ball.

It had been so long since I had really smiled, but the smile on my face this time was real. I was smiling on the inside, too. My hair and makeup were perfect, and I felt gorgeous. But most of all, I felt like I fit into the world I had never really known. I felt normal. At twenty-nine, a mother of two, I knew how lucky I was just to be alive. My confidence was sky-high, and I felt like a real woman. I knew what the mothers at that Mother's Day dance had felt like.

Finding the courage within yourself is so hard, but dreams and goals can be achieved. Sometimes you have to fight for them but you can never give up.

It's all about believing in yourself. I believed I could change, and I did—and now I feel I can do anything in life I want to. Believing is a gift of life.

My New Life

I have maintained my goal weight for eight years and I am so proud of myself. When I look at my reflection in the mirror today, I see a woman who is finally at peace with herself, a woman who has full control over her life, a woman who is content and so thankful and grateful for the life she has. I see so much love and happiness surrounding her. I thank God that woman is me.

My life is almost like some sort of fairy tale. Sometimes when I put my head down on my pillow at night, I'm almost too scared to go to sleep; I worry that when I wake everything will have snapped back to the way it used to be, that I'll be back to the obese me.

When I look back at my old life, it's as if I was a different person then, and in many ways I feel I've lived two lives. But I still ask some of the same questions I asked myself before I lost my weight, the same questions that plagued me in my old life. Questions like, why is all of this happening to me? Only now the answers to those questions have led me in a totally different direction—to help others lose the weight for good.

When I lost the weight, I had no one to turn to besides my husband, Jason. He was and still is my greatest supporter, but sometimes a husband or partner isn't enough. Husbands are supposed to say nice things. No matter what I weighed, Jason would always tell me he loved me regardless—and he meant it. I really appreciate that, of course, but I would have loved to have had someone else to listen to me, someone who had the same problem that I had, someone I could share my feelings and emotions with. Someone I could talk to and walk with, to motivate and encourage me, to cry and laugh with me. Back then I didn't know anyone who really understood my problem. All of the diets and diet centers I tried—and there were plenty—were staffed with people who'd never walked in my shoes. Skinny girls who'd lost a few pounds here or there, but had never had a serious weight problem. What would they know? And how would they know what it's like to be so fat you can't leave the house?

Now, I am that supporter. I am that person who listens and guides others through their journey. When I reached my goal weight I wanted everyone struggling with their weight to know that I could help. My story was featured in local newspapers, magazines and even television shows in Australia, and then I wrote *The Clothesline Diet* to share my diet program. It was a bestselling book and has become a source of inspiration for people all around the world. Every day I get letters from all corners of the globe—people telling me that they use my book to change their lives. It's a dream come true, and I get the most amazing sense of satisfaction from just being a shoulder to cry on or a friend to celebrate with. It goes to show, you never need to envy a success story because each and every one of us has a success story within—sometimes you just have to dig a little deeper to find it.

> *It's a dream come true to see other people shedding the weight that they've never before been able to shed.*

I'll never forget where I came from or the person I was. No matter how I look today on the outside, on the inside I am still the same Karen I was at 300 pounds. She is within my soul and I have so much to thank her for. Without her I wouldn't have had the chance to turn my life around. I wouldn't even have known that I have so much to give to others.

I believe that things happen for a reason, that we're all born with a destiny and that our past helps to shape our future. My weight loss has given me a second chance at life and now I make the most of every minute of every day. A few years ago, I used to have so much time on my hands I didn't know what to do with it, other than eat! Now, there aren't enough hours in the day to achieve everything I want to. There is so much possibility out there that I never knew existed when I was trapped inside my obesity shell. I'm like a child soaking up new experiences.

Not long ago, as I was doing my supermarket shopping, a lady approached me. She leaned over my cart and peered in to see what was there. She said to me, "You're her, aren't you? The clothesline woman." I smiled and before I could even mouth a yes she'd started rummaging through my cart! I couldn't believe how rude she was...until she explained that she was trying to lose weight. She picked up just about everything I had placed in the cart and was excitedly saying, "Oh, we can eat this. I didn't know I could have that." I was totally stunned!

We talked for forty-five minutes. She gave me a new insight into just how much of an impact my story has had on other people—everywhere. It's an incredible feeling to know that my diet plan works for other people, too; that gives me such a sense of satisfaction. I always knew that if it could work for me, it could work for anyone. But it's a dream come true to see other people shedding the weight that they've never before been able to shed and gaining the confidence to achieve things they never thought were possible.

One of my readers told an American friend, a doctor, about my story. She sent him a copy of *The Clothesline Diet*, and he invited me to help some of his patients in California.

Dr. Albert Bodt has opened up a new world to me and made me realize that obesity knows no borders. We had many discussions about how I lost my weight and what I was doing to help others do the same in Australia. He was so impressed by the simplicity of my plan and by my success that he invited me to come to his clinic in California and speak to his patients. What an honor! Now I travel to the U.S. regularly to help people lose weight and we're having great success, but there's still so much more work to be done. Americans spend $40 billion a year on diet books, products and weight-loss programs, so why then are 127 million Americans still overweight? America, it's time to shape up!

"Globesity" knows no borders. Weight loss doesn't require a passport, no matter what country or what state you are from, being overweight poses the same problems, creates the same heartache and requires the same dedication to overcome. You have everything at your fingertips to conquer obesity and

I'm going to help you do it. What you need now is a leader—someone who's walked in your shoes, who can show you the right path and cut through all of the crap. I am that person because I've been there, I've done it and I've succeeded. I know my story can change your life, so c'mon, America, let's get cracking! No more excuses. Together, we can win this battle. I may not be a health-care professional, I'm not a textbook expert, I haven't earned university degrees, but I've lived through obesity—every agonizing pound of it—and I've beaten it, and you can, too. In this book I share my story, warts 'n' all. I share my highs and lows, the same highs and lows you're probably going through right now. But most important, I give you the practical steps to create a whole new life—you already have all the tools. In this book you will find the inspirational story of how I overcame obesity, my tried-and-true seven-day diet plan, diet tips that *really* work and all the inspiration you need to make a fresh start.

You have everything at your fingertips to conquer obesity and I'm going to help you do it.

It only takes one step to change your life.

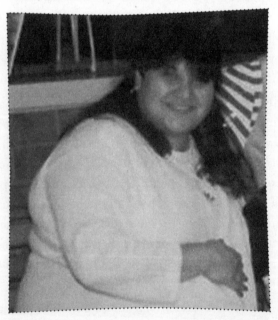

Before the Clothesline Diet

PART ONE

My Story

How I Lost 150 Pounds
and Changed My Life

CHAPTER ONE

The Heaviest Girl in the Class

AS LONG AS I CAN REMEMBER, I STRUGGLED WITH MY WEIGHT.
When I look back at photos of myself when I was as young as four years old,
I am the biggest girl at all of the parties. It was the same story at eight years
old, ten, twelve and so on. Nobody was the same size as me, nobody else was
in my shoes.

The pressure placed on an overweight child growing up is immense. The
peer pressure, pressure from your family and friends is subtle but constant,
and sometimes you feel as if you are being pounded from all sides. Everybody
stares at you, everybody talks behind your back and everybody feels sorry for
"the poor little fat girl." I was always that fat girl.

As an overweight child, that pressure is a terribly negative influence and
it really can have a lasting impact. It steers you toward an emotional dead end.
It makes you question your whole life.

I don't remember overeating or eating big meals as a child—I was just
always big. I can remember when I was in years five and six at primary school
and it came time for our school photos, the teachers would always put me in
the same spot. Back row, right in the middle. Even at that age I knew it was
because I was probably too big to fit anywhere else.

My real heartache, though, started on my first day of high school. I hadn't fit in with other kids my age at primary school, and I knew it would be no different at high school. I was embarrassed and nervous. I hardly knew most of the kids but I knew they would tease me, and I was so scared.

I was the biggest girl by far; I really stood out. Just getting my school uniform had been hard enough. Mum managed to buy the biggest size she could for me, but then she had to take all of the extra material off the hem and use it to add a panel at the back so I could fit into it. Everybody knew, and they would laugh at me for it. It was horrible.

I was vulnerable and very scared. Whenever the other kids made cruel comments, all I could do was take my parents' advice—ignore them and walk away. I could walk away, but I could not ignore what had been said. And each time I was taunted, the words would sink in a little more. Every day I would have to walk into that school. There was no escape; the thought of being there played on my mind all the time.

Each time I was taunted, the words would sink in a little more.

My relief from this was eating. The more I ate, the better I felt, and with every bite my problems just dissolved around me. Looking back, I realize that I couldn't control what I ate even then. It was my escape, my emotional crutch.

Taunted and Teased

Gym days every Wednesday were the worst—I'll never forget them. I used to complain to Mum and Dad that I was sick so I didn't have to go. Sometimes it worked and sometimes it didn't. I think they knew why I was "sick" so often.

When Mum and Dad did make me go on gym day, I would cry all the way to school because I knew that for the whole day I was going to get it from the other kids.

I couldn't control what I ate even then. It was my escape, my emotional crutch.

Sometimes our gym teacher would weigh us—that was a disaster. We would have to stand in front of the whole class while we were weighed. They called us out by name, and we had to walk up in front of the class and step on the scales. When we were on the scales our weight was called out to another teacher who noted it on our files.

There were enough people waiting in line close to the scales to hear the number called out. It didn't take long for news of my weight to spread around the class. I wanted to die—why was I so much fatter than all the other kids? What was wrong with me? While the other kids climbed, jumped rope and hung off the walls, I struggled and huffed and puffed my way through it; sometimes I couldn't do the activities at all. The kids would laugh at me and call me names like Humpty Dumpty and fat cat. Like I'd done in the morning, each gym day afternoon I would walk home in tears.

> *I wanted to die— why was I so much fatter than all the other kids?*

One day a boy in my class and some of his friends were sitting outside during recess. I walked by and one of the boys yelled out to me, "You fat dog, you fat ugly dog—what are you eating for lunch today?" All of his friends laughed at me.

I was so angry and embarrassed that I went into a rage. I rushed over with my fists up, ready to take him on and started to fight. I was almost in a trance. I was so upset that my mind and body were out of control. I actually picked him up and put his head through the classroom window! Afterward I saw the blood and I started screaming and crying. The other kids were shocked. The boy was taken to the hospital and had to have fifteen stitches.

> *The kids would laugh at me and call me names like Humpty Dumpty and fat cat.*

I ran all the way home and told Mum and Dad. In the meantime, the school had called. We all had to go back to face the principal. Mum and Dad acknowledged I'd done the wrong thing but they understood why. The school didn't. They put the blame on me.

I couldn't believe what I'd done or understand where my strength had come from, and I still can't believe it—what was I thinking? All I can say is that I really didn't mean to hurt that boy, but those comments had cut me to the core. I was so angry and so hurt by what he'd said that something just snapped inside me.

Word got around school to "look out for the fat girl" and things changed for the worse after that. I suffered through the year, but the final straw came one afternoon when I was beaten up as I was leaving school.

I'd barely gotten through the school gates when two girls lunged at me. The day before, they'd been waiting for me when I'd left the school and they'd stood by the gates yelling, "Fat girl, fat girl." I had ignored them up until then, but it was impossible to ignore them this afternoon.

The final straw came one afternoon when I was beaten up as I was leaving school.

They pushed me to the ground and while one kicked me in the stomach, the other punched me in the face. They were screaming at me—"Fat bitch!"—and I could feel blood running down the side of my head. They finally ran off, but by then the damage was done, physically and psychologically.

I headed straight back into school and found my teachers—they were horrified. Mum and Dad rushed up to the school and my teachers called the police. Mum just sobbed when she saw me. To my teachers, she cried, "How could you let this happen?"

I was very bruised and had cuts across my face, so there was no point trying to hide the beating. Mum and Dad drove me to and from school every day after that, and they took the school to court, but it was pointless—most of the damage done to me was inside my head.

It became too difficult to handle the ridicule and I pleaded with my parents to let me leave. After a lot of discussion, and a lot of persuasion from me, Mum and Dad begrudgingly agreed, but only on the condition that I got myself a job. I did just that and I left school before completing ninth grade, the day before my fifteenth birthday.

They were screaming at me—"Fat bitch!" —and I could feel blood running down the side of my head.

It was a sad experience because I really didn't want to miss out on an education and I had actually enjoyed schoolwork. But there was no way I could stay on after all the abuse.

By this point, I had already begun the diet roller coaster, not so much following a structured diet as going through periods of not eating to lose weight. I first started being conscious of what I ate and trying to starve myself when I was fourteen years old, primarily because of all the teasing I endured at school. I'd starve myself for two or three days and not have anything but water, until I started to feel faint and suffer dizzy spells. Then I'd pig out for the next few days and end up feeling so guilty that I'd starve again. It was a vicious roller coaster—and little did I realize that I'd be caught in that cycle for years to come.

The teasing didn't end with the students at my school, either. I can vividly remember one family dinner at a relative's house. At the time I'd just started going out with my first boyfriend, Robert. Everybody around the table knew I was trying to diet and that I was desperate to impress Robert. Instead of having a meal, I was eating a banana. As I peeled the skin back to eat it, one of my relatives snatched it out of my hand and squashed it inside a heavily buttered roll. She shoved it in my face and screeched, "Now eat!"

I first started being conscious of what I ate and trying to starve myself when I was fourteen years old.

All this happened in front of thirty relatives and my new boyfriend. I dropped the roll on the floor and ran outside crying. I was so ashamed. How could anyone be so cruel? I hid behind some trees in the garden, crying until Dad found me and took me home. I was only a teenager when this happened but it has remained etched in my memory.

That incident had a major impact on my life. Family are supposed to be the people you confide in and trust—they are supposed to love you unconditionally—but after that, I always wondered what my relatives were saying behind my back. All I could think was *if a relative could do something like that, imagine what everybody else is thinking about me.*

Trying for a Fresh Start

Leaving school and starting a new job was a turning point. I landed a job serving customers in a delicatessen at the local shopping center, and I was so excited. I counted down the days until I began. I thought that my first day at work would signal the end of torture. It was a new beginning and I was really proud.

As I expected, the first day was filled with excitement. I served customers, learned how to work the cash register and met some new people. By the time I got home I couldn't stop talking—I was ecstatic at how much I was learning.

On my second day, my boss taught me how to unpack boxes in the walk-in cooler out in back of the deli. That was great. Then the next day came and I was unpacking more boxes in the walk-in. And the next and the next day, I was still out in back. This had been going on for a while when I finally confronted my boss and asked her why I was always stuck in the walk-in. I spent so much time in there I was getting sick, developing colds. Being stuck in the dark all day meant I was drained of energy. She explained that that was where she wanted me to work and that that was where she needed me to be. Day after day I worked in that walk-in and every day I asked to be swapped with some other staff member serving out front.

My self-esteem started to wane and all of the doubts that had plagued me for so long came flooding back: she probably thinks I'm too fat to serve the customers. Maybe she thinks I'm going to eat all of the food out front. Or maybe she thinks I make a bad first impression. I pleaded with her one final time before she turned and snapped

> *My self-esteem started to wane and all of the doubts that had plagued me for so long came flooding back.*

at me. "Don't ask again, you're working there and that's that. Besides, you have enough fat on you to keep you warm anyway."

The rage that had come over me that day at school filled me again and I dragged her by the hair into the walk-in, shouting, "Let's see how long you'd like to stay in here for!" I locked her in, grabbed my things and left.

I never went back again. What a terror I was! But although there's no excuse for my behavior, she really had triggered a volatile mix of emotions— anger, shame, hurt and absolute despair.

It's hard to explain how I felt as an obese person. I lived with bitterness and anger on a daily basis. Looking back from where I am now, it really does feel like someone else's life, not mine.

Instead of wallowing I figured what had happened gave me the chance to fulfill one of my dreams—to work with children. So without any formal qualifications, I set off the next day looking for a job in child care. With a little luck, a lot of hard work and the help of my dad, who drove me everywhere, because I was only fifteen, I got the job I wanted.

> *I lived with bitterness and anger on a daily basis.*

We went door-to-door from one center to another. My lucky break came one afternoon when I walked into a child-care center in Sunshine, a suburb of Melbourne. The coordinator looked at me cautiously before asking what I wanted. "A job," I replied. We talked about my skills and I explained that I didn't have formal qualifications but did a lot of work at home and helped Mum look after my younger brother and sister. The coordinator agreed to take me on. I was ecstatic when she offered me a job on the spot—straightaway she introduced me to the other staff and the children.

I was to start the following Monday and the days dragged as I waited. I was so excited, I just wanted to start my job.

On Monday morning I turned up forty-five minutes early and worked alongside Sylvia, one of the caregivers, for the first week to learn the children's routines. They made me feel important and needed. I hadn't felt like that before. Three out of the five women who worked there were large and I was comfortable being there and being around them.

As the weeks went by I assisted with each age group, working with new staff members along the way. The girls were fantastic and I became good friends with them. I admired them because they were almost as large as me, but it didn't seem to affect them. They treated their weight as though it wasn't an issue. Working with them and the children distracted my thoughts from my own weight. I could really be myself and the people I met gave me a lot of confidence.

My naked body reflected back at me made me cringe.

After I'd been there six weeks I was told I could have a group of children on my own. This was such a great feeling: I was really proud. I was going to be looking after the three- and four-year-olds.

At work my life couldn't have been better. I treated those children like they were my own, although in reality I was still a child myself—I hadn't even turned sixteen. Each night after dinner I would sit in my room and plan everything I would do with the children the next day. I was totally absorbed in my job and I loved it.

There was a small downfall, though. Every morning I would still have to see myself in the bathroom mirror. I would wake up full of enthusiasm and rush into the shower to get ready for work, and there it was—my naked body reflected back at me made me cringe. Once I saw the children's smiling faces, though, all of the anguish would disappear.

A Constant Struggle

Looking back, I realize there was always a battle going on in my mind, with part of me thinking I should accept myself and get on with life and the other part believing I was a total disgrace.

In some ways I believed my only real best friend at that time was a hamburger, hot dog or cream bun. After eating something like that, I knew it would stay with me forever and keep me comforted on my stomach, legs or bottom. Food would never leave me like friends or boyfriends might. Along with these thoughts, though, I felt I was being enslaved by food, that it was overpowering me.

No matter where I turned for help, food was staring at me with its devilish power of possession. Many times I begged Mum to help me lose weight. She would say to me, "But, Karen, what is the use of cooking healthy food at home when you go out and fill yourself up with junk?" And she was right. If I went out with friends I would inevitably end up stuffing my face with rubbish.

I felt I was being enslaved by food, that it was over-powering me.

Whenever I went out for dinner, I was always the last to order because I was so paranoid that I would over order. If I ordered more than the others at the table I was ashamed. In front of other people I would eat tiny portions of food and starve all night rather than be seen eating too much. But, of course, when I got home I would head straight to the fridge and eat everything I could get my hands on. I'd stuff myself until I felt sick. And I would always pile on another pound or two doing so.

If only I could have known then how different life can be.

By the time I was sixteen I weighed 180 pounds and I was very depressed. The type of depression and sadness you feel when someone close to you dies—that was how I felt almost all of the time.

It's strange to reflect on those teenage days. I should have had a happy life—a great family, including wonderful parents, and all the opportunity in the world. And yet, I didn't have the body or the inner confidence to really be myself. So much of me was shielded by my weight. I used it to hide from the real world. If only I could have known then how different life can be.

"I have a new lease on life."

Rosetta

Starting Weight: **183** pounds

Current Weight: **125** pounds

58 POUNDS LOST!

After I gave birth to my twins, my nurse told me I needed to lose weight. That was sixteen years and a lot of diets ago. But I've finally achieved my goal. I've lost nearly 60 pounds since starting Karen's program. I'd been wanting to lose a few pounds, but I didn't think I was too badly overweight. But I went along to Karen's group to keep a friend company and as I started to lose weight I was feeling better and better about myself; that's when I knew I really had been too big. The more weight I lost the healthier I felt. I had more energy and I was much happier: I had a new lease on life! People didn't recognize me. I now wish I'd done it years ago. It took me a year to lose all the weight, but it's changed my life and I love being able to buy clothes off the rack now. Losing weight was really hard work, but I believe now that I've achieved this I can achieve anything.

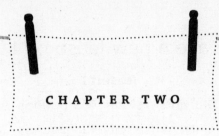

CHAPTER TWO

Wedding Belle Blues

WHEN I WAS FIFTEEN, MY COUSIN ASKED IF I WANTED TO GO TO her school dance. I looked forward to that night and made a special effort to look good. I had my hair permed, bought new makeup to hide my chubby face, and bought a beautiful loose pink silk shirt that hid the ripples of fat on my back and around my waist. I felt pretty.

We danced and danced all night. But out of the corner of my eye I noticed a guy paying us a lot of attention. He was leaning up against a wall just staring at us while we danced. We stopped to get a drink and he followed us over and bought me one. He was really cute and looked much older than the teenagers at the dance.

We stopped and talked for hours—this guy just had me under a spell. His name was Michael. We were together for the rest of the dance and by then he had totally swept me off my feet. I gave him my phone number and I desperately hoped I'd be seeing him again.

The very next morning, much to my surprise, he phoned me and from that day we began a relationship. My parents warned me about him, they didn't like him right from the start, but I was young and in love and didn't care. I now believe I was just craving affection, and so I fell head over heels for anyone who showed me the slightest bit of attention.

Falling in Love

Michael and I stayed together for three years, and there was a time when I actually thought he would be the man I married—how wrong I was! He was quite a private person but I had no reason not to trust him. Often he would go off on his own and I never questioned where he was going or what he was doing.

But when we started talking about getting engaged, I wanted to know more about what he was up to. Inevitably, when I quizzed him he would become very aggressive and sometimes he even slapped me in the face to keep me quiet. It worked. And despite the abuse, not once did I ever stop loving him.

It was the most humiliating time for me. I felt gutted. I cried for weeks on end.

Our engagement plans were all in place and the wedding date set when Michael suddenly disappeared. I thought he might have had last-minute nerves, or maybe was planning a surprise for me. But for days I didn't hear a thing from Michael. I was distraught, I didn't know what had happened to him—if he was alive or dead, or if he'd simply left me. I was an emotional wreck.

I spent days phoning people, trying to find him, until one of his friends finally confessed that he was hiding out at his friend Jason's house. I stormed over to confront him, and he explained that he wasn't ready for commitment and that our relationship was over.

It was the most humiliating time for me. I felt gutted. I cried for weeks on end. I thought that Michael would be the answer to all of my problems. He'd supported me when I left school and he'd made me forget all about my weight and the negative emotions I was battling with each day.

I lay in bed believing that no one would ever love me. Of course, I turned to my old friend— food—for comfort.

Our breakup made me feel like such a failure. I convinced myself that it was my fault he'd run off, and for many nights I lay in bed believing I had no future and that no one would ever love me. Of course, I turned to my old friend—food—for comfort.

Months later I happened to bump into Michael's friend Jason again. Of course we got chatting about Michael. It turned out Jason and Michael had fallen out and we now shared a dislike for him. From the moment I met Jason again, something clicked. He seemed so kind and compassionate. We seemed to run into each other often, and eventually Jason asked me out.

He was very romantic and very different from anybody I'd ever met before. Not once did he ever comment about my weight or look sideways at me; it just wasn't an issue. And if anybody dared to make the smallest gesture to me about it, he was on to them straightaway.

We had come together for mutual comfort, but it wasn't long before things changed. Jason and I really enjoyed our time together and fell in love very quickly. So much so that five months after we started going out we got engaged. We were just seventeen and eighteen when we decided to marry.

> *We were putting on weight without even knowing it.*

Jason was incredibly hardworking—he has always been very ambitious—and was in the fourth year of his apprenticeship as a machinist. He put in a lot of effort to build a stable career and often told me of his hopes to create a comfortable future for his family. My parents accepted Jason from the first time they met him.

It was these qualities that made him so appealing. I felt like I was really set for life with Jason by my side.

Letting Out the Wedding Dress, Again and Again

When I look back now it seems funny that when I first got together with Jason I never worried about what food I ate or how much I weighed. I had well and truly tipped 180 pounds on the scales around the time we met, and Jason weighed about 187 pounds.

One night, about six months after we first started seeing each other, we began talking about our weight, and decided to weigh ourselves. Jason weighed 198 pounds and I weighed 183 pounds. I remember it vividly. We were putting on weight without even knowing it, but even then we did nothing about it. We often went out for dinner dates, and we loved to go to the beach and eat fish and chips while watching the sun go down. It wasn't great for our waistlines, but we were happy.

It was mid-August when we began planning our engagement party, but after hours of talking through our ideas, Jason suggested, "Let's just get married instead."

We were very young, but I loved Jason so much. Jason accepted me totally. He loved me for who I was, for my personality, not for my weight or how I looked. And he made me feel really good about myself. I knew in my heart it would work out, so I agreed.

My parents offered to turn their garage into a bungalow for us so we could live there while we saved up for our first house. It also meant they could keep watch over us to make sure everything was okay.

A week later we had a private engagement celebration, then began full preparations for our big day. I was so excited. Everything was carefully organized: the cake, the rings, cars and dresses.

My weight naturally became an issue again when I was shopping for my wedding dress. I carefully chose the times I went into shops; I'd go either early in the morning or late in the afternoon when I hoped there'd be fewer people around.

Within a matter of weeks of announcing our plans to marry, I began to pile on pounds like there was no tomorrow.

Within a matter of weeks of announcing our plans to marry, I began to pile on pounds like there was no tomorrow. Most brides shed them—but not me! My weight ballooned to 231 pounds. I'd put on nearly 50 pounds in six months! I hated walking into bridal salons—absolutely hated it—and as the time of our wedding got closer I became quite reclusive.

I tried on scores of dresses before I finally found the one I wanted to wear. The dress was amazing: it was covered with sequins and had a train that was three yards long and a veil that was four. It was huge—and so was I!

I felt like a princess while I was wearing it.

The biggest size the dress came in was 24 and it had to be ordered in. The day it arrived I got to the shop as quickly as I could, I was so excited. I took the dress off the hanger and squeezed myself into the change room. The dress was tight across my chest and I could barely do the zipper at the back—I burst into tears. The shop assistant was lovely; she suggested that as the wedding was twelve weeks away, if I hadn't lost any weight in six weeks' time, they could get the dress altered.

I really tried hard. I was determined that I would lose some weight, but after two weeks I became distracted. My old eating habits soon returned, except that I ate more than ever before.

With five weeks to go until the wedding, it was time for me to have a final fitting of the dress. Well, this time the zipper wouldn't even budge—I'd packed on more weight. My dress had to be sent out to be resized—made bigger! Can you imagine how fat I was?

By the time the dress was finally ready it was perfect, but two weeks before the big day I tried it on again, and it wouldn't fit, I'd put on even more weight. Thankfully a friend, who was also making my headdress, told me that she could fix it, and sure enough off it went again to be enlarged, arriving back with just two days to spare.

It was my wedding day. It was supposed to be the happiest day of my life, and here I was, sobbing, disgusted with, and deeply disappointed in, myself because I couldn't lose any weight.

By the time the day arrived, April 21, 1990, I was awash with nerves—my dress was spread out on Mum and Dad's bed—it nearly covered the entire bed and could've doubled as a bedspread. When I got out of the shower that morning the first thing I did was jump on the scales. The numbers flicked around in front of my face before the scales finally settled at 256 pounds.

It really hit me how big I was. I closed the bathroom door and sat alone, crying my eyes out. It was my wedding day. It was supposed to be the happiest day of my life, and here I was, sobbing. I was so disgusted with, and deeply disappointed in, myself because I couldn't lose any weight.

I sat for a while until my tears subsided, then continued to get myself ready. I put on a brave face in front of everyone, smiling like a radiant bride should.

Our wedding went off without a hitch; it was everything I dreamed it would be. Throughout the ceremony I felt like a princess and everyone told me how beautiful I looked.

But as we walked into the reception my weight was staring back at me—there were mirrors all around the room and I whispered to Jason, "My God, look how fat I am!"

I was suddenly petrified that we wouldn't fit through the bridal arch together. We'd have to go through one at a time! As we walked past all of our guests my heart started pumping—how embarrassing it would be if we couldn't get through! We reached the arch and Jason moved his shoulders slightly ahead of me—very cunningly we managed to squeeze through and nobody ever knew my dilemma.

Wedded Bliss...and Wedded Blues

Our honeymoon to Fiji was our first real chance to be on our own; it was a fantastic experience. But even on our honeymoon, my weight was always at the back of my mind. Our room had the most magnificent view of the swimming pool below and we couldn't wait to get in there, but I insisted that we go down when it was getting dark because I didn't want people staring at me in my swimsuit.

We made the most of that time. While we were on our honeymoon, Jason and I decided we wanted to start a family. We tried day and night—and had a lot of fun doing it! But even though we were trying for children, there were parts of my body that I would not let Jason touch. It's bizarre—I was married to the man I loved so much and so intimately, the person I trusted with my life, and yet I wouldn't let him touch my stomach. I was so paranoid about my weight I begged him not to touch me, and I put up a wall in my mind around parts of my body. I visualized the wall and he wasn't allowed to go behind it—that was private.

I was married to the man I loved so much and so intimately, and yet I wouldn't let him touch my stomach.

By the time we were leaving, I was convinced I was pregnant. The week had flown by and we couldn't wait to get home and tell everyone that we were trying to have a baby.

We'd been back from Fiji for about three weeks and I still hadn't had my period. I was very excited—I was sure I was pregnant. I rushed out to the drugstore one afternoon and bought a home pregnancy test kit. I did it three times, but each time it showed up negative. I didn't believe the results and assumed it was too early in my pregnancy for a positive result to register.

A week later my period still hadn't arrived so I made an appointment at the doctor's to have a blood test—it showed up negative, too. Jason and I couldn't understand why the results were negative because we were so certain I was carrying our baby.

It was at that time the doctor mentioned that I should consider losing some weight. I was about 264 pounds and I knew I had to do something about it—my doctor told me my weight would make it very difficult for me to conceive.

In the car coming home I told Jason that I was going on a diet. It wasn't a particularly new revelation; he'd heard the same promise many times before. The daily pigging out on junk food—like pizzas and the midnight family block of chocolate that had become a normal part of my diet—had to stop. The pounds were adding up at this stage and the only real explanation was that Jason and I were so happy with one another and our life together that

> *I was 264 pounds and I knew I had to do something about it.*

until then we'd been oblivious to it. But I was desperate to start a family and I knew the only way that could happen would be if I lost some of my weight. I dieted off and on, but nothing worked.

This went on for two and a half years, and not one day during that time did we stop trying to conceive. I got more and more depressed that I wasn't getting pregnant. And although I was supposed to be losing weight, I sought comfort in food. The more depressed I became,

> *I sought comfort in food. The more depressed I became, the more of a comfort food became; it was a vicious cycle.*

the more of a comfort food became; it was a vicious cycle that didn't stop. My doctor really pressed me to lose some weight and to concentrate on what I ate. Well, for me concentrating on food was like an invitation to eat!

We had sporadic bursts of hope and when I thought I could be pregnant. I'd rush off to the drugstore and buy the home pregnancy test, fingers crossed, hoping for the best—but the results were always negative.

Both Jason and I were at our lowest and our lives had changed. I found it difficult to make love to Jason. Often in the middle of making love I would push him away, burst into tears and run out of the room. Some nights I'd go out driving in the car and would be gone for hours while I calmed myself down.

I tried to explain to Jason that I didn't think we could live as husband and wife if we couldn't have a child. I just couldn't wake up every morning pretending nothing was wrong when this was a big issue in our lives. Jason was constantly telling me he loved me and that we would work through our problems together, but I had different thoughts in my head. I convinced myself that he couldn't love me. I kept feeling he deserved a wife who could give him children. Often, we ended up in huge fights.

It was my fault our dreams couldn't come true—it was all because I couldn't lose weight.

Even before we were married it had been our goal to have children, and from the first day we became husband and wife, it was the biggest thing in our lives. To have that dream ripped out from under you is shattering. I blamed myself. It was my fault our dreams couldn't come true—it was all because I couldn't lose weight.

It seemed that IVF was our only option. We met with specialists who told us that through IVF we had a 12 percent chance of having a child. I felt our future together was hanging on a 12 percent chance. Often we asked ourselves, how much worse can our lives get, how low can we go?

The more I tried to lose weight, the more obsessed I became with eating.

I knew our failure to conceive was because of my weight. All the doctors and specialists we saw said the same thing—"You're overweight." We had to wait twelve months before we could start IVF and I thought that time would allow me to shed the pounds.

I tried harder than ever to lose weight, and I did—but every time I lost two pounds, the next week I'd put three back on. I just couldn't lose it. My weight wouldn't budge.

Our inability to have a child became the focus of our lives and the issue that caused the most problems. Jason tried to cheer me up; some nights he'd pack a picnic and take me down to the beach for dinner. He was incredibly considerate. But as we'd walk beside the water, I'd see parents playing with their children and that would upset me all over again.

That year waiting for IVF was hellish. We often tried to lose weight and we'd be good for one day, then eat pizza the next. The more I tried to lose weight, and the more I wanted to, the more obsessed I became with eating.

I ate for any reason at all, but mainly out of habit. I don't know why it was so hard for me when I wanted to have a baby so badly, but it was. Something within me needed to change but my self-esteem was so low it was impossible for me to motivate myself.

Jason suggested we look into finding some new hobbies to do together to take our minds off waiting for IVF. We put a darts team together and bought an old trailer that we refurbished as a weekend hobby. At night, though, when we lay in bed, all of our troubles came flooding back and often I would cry myself to sleep. There were so many questions that nobody could answer for me. Why was I unable to have a child? Was I being punished for being fat? Jason could hear me crying and I knew he was awake, too. I pulled him down with me. He was trying to be strong, and I dragged him into my depression.

Statistically, the chances of our getting pregnant were very low. Due to my increased weight and poor health, our odds of getting pregnant with IVF were as low as 2.5 percent. It didn't give us a lot of hope! But despite the doctor's warning that it might not be successful, when the day finally came around for us to be implanted—I could hardly wait. I was so excited! Jason was a little more reserved, and he reminded me to keep calm and wait for a few weeks to make sure everything was okay with the pregnancy. He was worried that I would be let down again if I got overexcited—honestly, though, nothing could have dampened my spirits or calmed me down. But while in my heart I hoped for the best, I also knew I had to prepare myself for the worst, just in case.

The doctor warned us that I had to rest, really rest. In two weeks the results would come back to tell us if the IVF had been a success. Those two weeks seemed to take forever. All we could do was sit there and hope.

The day the results came back, both our parents stayed with me for the day. They paced up and down the backyard and sat by the phone—they made me even more nervous. By the time Jason got home from work, the clinic still hadn't rung and I was desperate to find out if I was carrying our baby. I was getting edgier and edgier by the minute, and eventually I said to Jason, "I just can't wait any longer—I'm ringing them." I went to the toilet to calm my nerves before I made the phone call, and in the space of a minute my world came crashing down. I found blood.

I was numb; I sat on the toilet in disbelief.

Finally I got myself together and walked out, but Jason knew something was wrong straightaway. My tongue seized up and my mouth was dry. Jason was asking me what was wrong and I couldn't speak. He nagged and nagged at me before I finally managed to open my mouth and tell him I had my period.

We were both shattered. This was the very day we had been hoping to hear the best news of our lives—and we were let down again. Jason tried to reassure me and encouraged me to call the clinic anyway. He was trying to keep me calm and was rubbing my hand, but I needed to make the call on my own.

I took a few big deep breaths and picked up the phone. I explained to the nurse what had just happened. She said that sometimes women bleed in the first couple of weeks of pregnancy and told me not to worry while she went and grabbed my file. That eased my mind a little and I felt a tiny flicker of hope. But my heart was beating fast and I had cramps in my stomach from nerves. When she came back to the phone, the tone of her voice had changed and become much more serious. She said to me, "Karen, I'm so sorry but the tests have come back negative."

This was the very day we had been hoping to hear the best news of our lives—and we were let down again.

I couldn't speak; I just hung up. My mouth was tight and dry, and I felt sick.

I will never forget that day—the memories are vivid. I just let go there and then, all of the pressure that had built up as I waited just burst from inside me.

I managed to give the impression that I was coping well in the months that followed. I still smiled and laughed, and I seemed happy. But on the inside I felt like my whole world had imploded. I hated myself more and more, and I just stopped caring about my weight—I didn't care about my life. I thought that if I couldn't have our baby there was no purpose for me on this earth.

There were days that I didn't even bother to brush my hair; I was struggling just to get out of bed. It was as though I were sinking in quicksand, and every now and then Jason would grab me and lift me out, but the quicksand was faster than he was.

It just seemed that having a family was not meant to be for us. We had tried everything, and nothing had worked. So together we decided to save our money, put it toward our house and make that the focus of our lives.

We found the perfect plot of land and began building our dream house. It was just around the corner from Mum and Dad's and we walked past it every day, watching it grow. Building the house gave me a purpose and the day we finally got the keys I was ecstatic. That night we made love in our own bed in our new home, and we felt like our lives were finally turning for the better.

The Beginning of the End

I'd begun to see a little more of an old friend—Melissa. We'd go out for coffee and talk on the phone and Jason was quite friendly with her husband. We spent a lot of time together and whenever I wasn't at home, Jason would always find me at Melissa's house. I was actually spending more time with her than with Jason, which was putting a lot of pressure on our relationship, but I felt free with her. I think I was just desperately lonely. Often Jason would work the night shift, so Melissa would come and keep me company or I'd stay with her.

But then she started paying a lot more attention to Jason. She told me Jason had been calling her from work, confiding our marital problems and she was helping him. I began to become very suspicious of her motives but kept thinking *she's my best friend, she wouldn't do anything*. Despite my rationalizations, I could see things happening between them, in their body language and the little phrases and things they'd say to one another. I had the sinking suspicion that something was going on.

I felt utterly betrayed by my husband and my best friend.

Then one night at a party at our place I overheard her telling him, "You can do better, Jason," and as I went to confront them they kissed. I was stunned. I felt utterly betrayed by my husband and my best friend. Jason denied anything was going on, but I felt incredibly torn. I didn't know how I could ever trust him again.

Jason swore it was the first time they'd ever kissed, and for weeks we talked and argued about what had happened. I loved him so much and I desperately wanted to stay married. He convinced me that he loved me and tried to convince me that everything was okay, but my mind was in a state of turmoil. Of course, I turned to my old pal food for comfort.

This went on for weeks and weeks, until one night Jason and I were at home alone watching TV. We hadn't made love in months, not since I saw them kissing. Jason liked to lie on the floor on a mattress to help his sore back and this night I was feeling sympathetic, so I offered to give him a back rub. I told him to take his shirt off and I started rubbing some massage oil into his back.

His skin felt soft and warm, and while I was rubbing him I was overcome by feelings and started to cry. He asked me what was wrong and I didn't know—I think I was scared, scared of losing him and our marriage.

My hands were full of massage oil and I rubbed it into his chest and we kissed. The only lights on in the house were the Christmas lights. We kissed and kissed in the darkness. There was so much passion between us, my heart was pounding and I was sweating. He was so gentle with me and he made me forget about my insecurities. He made me feel beautiful.

My weight didn't enter my mind and the problems of not having a baby were suddenly so far away. Nothing was important at that moment apart from loving Jason. It was almost like the first night we'd ever made love. Afterward, I began to sob again. I didn't want to lose the love that we had and I feared in my heart that our relationship, our marriage, would never be the same.

Over the next couple of months, Jason and I tried to make things work, but things were always tense between us. We had created a wall and it seemed impossible to tear it down. Everything came to a head during a Christmas party I threw that year. As a gesture of a goodwill, I invited Melissa and her husband. As I was serving food and drinks, I caught Jason and Melissa in another moment: Jason was walking inside through the sliding door just as Melissa stepped out, and they hesitated there, face-to-face, their bodies touching, until Melissa brushed Jason's hip to move past him.

My heart sank; I was absolutely crushed. And I knew then that no matter how much I loved Jason and wanted to make our marriage work, it was simply not going to be possible.

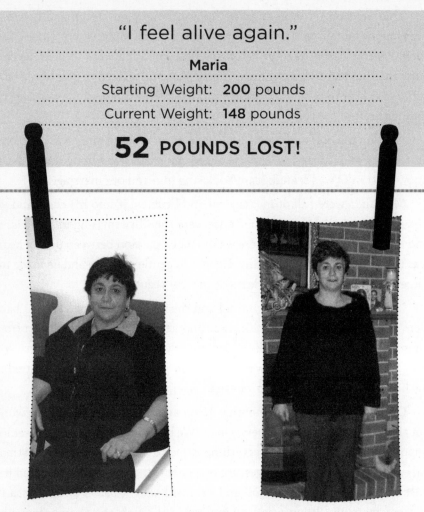

"I feel alive again."

Maria

Starting Weight: **200** pounds

Current Weight: **148** pounds

52 POUNDS LOST!

I wanted to lose weight because I was sick of people thinking I was pregnant all the time. I felt that people were always staring at me because I was so big. I was tired of wearing pants with elastic and not being able to fit into boots. I wanted to be able to fit into some nice clothes for once. Clothes looked awful on me and I didn't have the energy to exercise.

I'd never really thought about going to a weight-loss group before because I was quite depressed and I didn't think I'd fit in. I felt that life was just passing me by.

Then I saw Karen on TV and she changed my attitude. She made me believe that I could lose weight. Through *The Clothesline Diet*, she taught me how to eat healthy food and maintain my weight. I have read all of her books and they have inspired me to achieve my ideal weight. They are like a bible to me.

Now I have a great time shopping for clothes—and I can fit comfortably into a size 12. I am more active and less self-conscious. People who never spoke to me before take the time to talk to me now and tell me how great I look. I feel alive again.

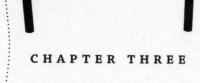

CHAPTER THREE

My Little Miracle

YET AGAIN, THERE WAS ONE LOYAL FRIEND I TURNED TO FOR comfort. Food. And lots of it. I really started to gain more weight after our breakup. I was big before but this was a major turning point in my life—unfortunately, for the worse.

I ate and ate and ate. Snacks were actually a banquet. Late at night I thought about our breakup; that was my worst time. Late-night feasts became a daily occurrence. I'd eat a whole package of scones, followed by six or seven granola bars and maybe a grilled sandwich before I went to bed. I was really ballooning, but the food gave me comfort so I couldn't stop.

There was one loyal friend I turned to for comfort. Food. And lots of it.

Christmas Eve was terrible. Normally we would have had both our families together and I would have cooked dinner, but this year I sat on the couch watching television and crying. My cousins were heading to the beach for a few days after New Year's. I didn't really want to go but Mum insisted I should. My cousins and I talked all the way there in the car, but once we had arrived, they made a rule that we were not to speak Jason's name for the rest of the week. At first I thought I couldn't do it, but then I agreed that it was probably a good idea.

I thought about Jason a lot and I rang home every day to see if he'd called or if anyone had seen him. Always after these calls I'd become quiet and go off on my own for a while. Whenever I felt down, my cousins made me laugh, or took me out to take my mind off my problems. They were a great comfort to me.

I started to feel unwell while I was away, but assumed it was just tiredness. I'd been under a lot of stress, I wasn't sleeping and I wasn't eating well, and it was starting to take its toll. But by the time I got home, Mum was adamant that I was going to see a doctor and she made me an appointment for the next day.

The first thing the doctor did was take my blood pressure—it was very high. I explained to him what I'd been going through, and he said that my symptoms were probably due to stress. But my periods had been acting up, too. This happened quite often because of my weight, but I hadn't had a period for two months. He asked me if there was any chance I could be pregnant and I just laughed. I said, "No—I wish." To be certain he suggested doing a pregnancy test anyway. He looked at me and said, "This is really strange. This test isn't showing negative or positive—I think you should have a further blood test."

It was the happiest day of my life, and yet overwhelmingly sad at the same time.

Mum's face just lit up, but I told her not to get her hopes up. I said to the doctor, "Look, this is wasting your time and my time." But he insisted.

Wednesday came and the results were due, so I rang the clinic, fully expecting to be let down again. The nurse at the clinic told me the doctor wanted me to come in, rather than give me the results over the phone. My first thought was that I must have had an infection, and Mum and I went back to the clinic again.

We sat down, and he said, "Karen... congratulations, you're pregnant."

Mum started jumping up and down, screaming and crying—while I ran to the toilet to be sick. I was so shocked—I just couldn't believe it was true. When I came out, Mum was hugging the doctor.

The night I had conceived was the last night Jason and I had made love in our new house. So many questions flooded my mind. How could I tell Jason? What would he say? What would he think?

It was the happiest day of my life, and yet overwhelmingly sad at the same time. We had dreamed of this day for so long and now Jason wasn't here to share it with me. I needed to tell him. I'd been longing for years to have this conversation with him, but now I hardly knew how to pick up the phone. It had been about four weeks since I'd seen Jason, and I was very excited and nervous, anticipating the expression on his face when I told him I was pregnant.

I went around to his parents' place at four o'clock that same day. I knew he'd be home from work then and I was determined he would hear it from me—nobody else. He opened the door and when I told him we needed to talk, he just stared at me blankly. The bitterness he felt toward me was obvious.

We agreed to go to our house to talk. We walked inside and sat down, and he offered me coffee. He was very blunt and seemingly totally devoid of emotion. He said to me flatly, "Okay, you've got me here—what did you want to talk about?"

I began to explain that I'd been to the doctor earlier that day, and he'd told me I was two months pregnant.

I wasn't expecting the reaction I got.

Deep down I'd hoped it would prompt a reunion, but instead he was furious. It was a side of him that I'd never seen before. He didn't believe I was pregnant and, worse, he didn't believe the baby was his since we'd tried for so long and failed. He asked me how they could prove I was pregnant—and I told him that I'd had a blood test. He didn't believe me and insisted that I have another blood test done while he was present. I agreed and told him to choose a doctor, pick a time and date and that I would be there. I gave him our family doctor's card in case he wanted to talk to him in the meantime, but he ripped it up in my face.

> *He didn't believe I was pregnant and, worse, he didn't believe the baby was his.*

Jason thought I was using a phantom pregnancy as a ploy for us to get back together, and although I longed to be back in Jason's arms, I certainly didn't fall pregnant to trap him! A few weeks later a letter arrived from his lawyer requesting a DNA test to prove the baby was actually his. That was a real low point in my life. I knew who the father was but the fact that Jason doubted me showed how much the trust between us had broken down.

Jason's lawyer wanted me to have the DNA test while I was pregnant, which meant an injection into my stomach that risked harm to the baby—there was no way I would agree to this. He'd just have to wait until the baby was born.

Life on My Own

Months went by and I didn't see Jason at all. I couldn't bear the thought of Jason living in our dream house without me, and we agreed to sell the house we'd worked so hard to build. All this time, I'd thought Jason and I would be able to reconcile, but now I was on my own and pregnant. Deep down I missed Jason enormously, and I loved him wholeheartedly, but the reality was that he just wasn't with me.

The day of our fifth wedding anniversary arrived, and I sat by the phone desperately hoping he would call. But he didn't. I lay in bed that night wondering what he did on our anniversary day, and I rubbed my growing stomach and talked to my baby. Oh, and I ate!

Although there were a lot of negative things going on in my life, the baby made life worth living and I often comforted myself by talking to my stomach.

My weight really packed on, and as each week went by and the pounds went up so did my blood pressure. By the time I was five months pregnant and had to have a biweekly checkup, it was getting worse each visit. Some nights I'd have to stay in the hospital and be monitored, but funnily enough I never felt alone. I had the baby with me and I began to come to terms with having the baby on my own.

Eight months into the pregnancy my blood pressure was far too high and I was admitted into the hospital. I spent days there, trying to bring it down. I was monitored constantly. I had weekly checkups and each time I took my bags with me because I'd spend a few nights there. I couldn't believe that Jason didn't get in contact with me through all this. I was a little sad about it, but I also had a new uplifting focus—the baby inside me. I visualized

I ate everything in sight—I couldn't stop eating. And I was huge.

loving this baby, holding him and rocking him. I lived for the baby to come and I thanked God he gave me a reason for being on this earth.

My baby and my family were all I had to live for.

About three and a half weeks before I was due, my weight ballooned to 282 pounds. I ate everything in sight—I couldn't stop eating. And I was huge.

I spent the last month of my pregnancy in my brother's bedroom, and Mum would feed me constantly, telling me I was eating for two—which I know now is very wrong! But it was a great excuse to eat more.

My blood pressure became dangerously high. My legs and feet were so swollen they looked like they would burst, my hands were full of fluid and, to top it off, the baby pressed on one of the nerves in my right leg, all but paralyzing me. I couldn't walk. I was just too big and it was too uncomfortable. I had to grab one of Mum and Dad's bar stools to lean on and drag my leg behind me everywhere I went. I used it as a walker.

No matter what position I was in, I was too big to get comfortable and the pain in my leg was unbearable. At two or three in the morning I'd scream out in pain and Mum would rub my legs for me. With two weeks to go I had another checkup and the doctors could see I was in pain, so they booked me in for a special massage to see if the baby would move off that spot. It didn't—I had no choice but to put up with the pain until the baby decided to arrive.

I shed a lot of tears in those last weeks. I was happy that I was pregnant but I didn't think it was fair I was in so much pain. The quicker the baby came the better it would be.

I knew my baby was in danger because of my blood pressure. For the last two weeks I lived on the couch and didn't move except to go to the toilet, and I knew that when I had to go it was going to be hideous. I'd call out to my parents in incredible pain and they tried to help me walk to the toilet. It was a family effort; Dad helped me up while Mum picked up my legs and helped me take each step. I kept focusing on the thought that it would all be worth it when the baby came.

In those final weeks I missed Jason a lot. He was on my mind constantly, especially since I knew we were having our baby soon and I hadn't seen him. Maybe it was just because I was becoming a mother, but I really wanted him near me. He never made any effort to get in touch with me, not even a quick call to ask how I was doing, and that caused me a lot of grief. I knew he had doubts in his mind but surely a part of him was wondering if the baby was his.

Welcoming My Miracle into the World

As my due date approached, my blood pressure was still high. My doctor was very concerned, and wanted to book me into the hospital to rest and be monitored again for a few days. He told me my blood pressure was so high there was a danger it would poison my placenta. So the decision was made to induce me.

They strapped a baby monitor on me, stimulated contractions and broke my water. I managed to sleep that night and by the next morning I was feeling a small amount of pain but nothing significant. The doctors encouraged me to get out of bed and walk around the hospital. Hours and hours passed and by nine o'clock that night, there was still no progress. I was feeling pain, but I was so fat there was no position I could get comfortable in.

Brendan was my miracle. Every ounce of heartbreak I'd been through was worth it.

That's when the pain started to increase. I cried out for an epidural and they gave me two shots, but I was so big they couldn't find the right spot! By one o'clock, I was still in pain, and the baby's heart rate dropped. I was crying and screaming to the nurses, "I can't stand this anymore—please, make it happen!" Within seconds the baby's heart rate dipped dangerously low and, before I knew what was happening, I was rushed for an emergency cesarean. I begged them not to let my baby die—he was all I had in life.

It only took about three minutes before they lifted the baby out and presented him to me, saying, "Congratulations, Karen, you've got a baby boy."

I cried. My mum was sobbing; the joy, the excitement. I desperately wanted to hold him but they took him away to be washed. Mum said to me, "Oh, Karen—he looks so much like Jason." And he did—he still does today.

At that moment, I wished Jason were at my side. I was happy to have Mum there but I desperately wanted my husband, the father of our child. This moment was something we had dreamed of for so long. He had missed his son being born and he could never get the moment back.

They cleaned the baby up and handed him back to me. I called him Brendan Lee. Brendan was my miracle. Every ounce of heartbreak I'd been through was worth it. I was a mum—and if I had to do it all again, I would without missing a beat. Brendan weighed seven pounds seven ounces—a beautiful, healthy little bundle, and to me nothing else in the world mattered.

The nurses took him back and sent me to my room to rest. They bathed him and weighed him while my parents and brother and sister looked on.

The pain I'd felt a few hours before had disappeared. By five o'clock in the morning, the nurses asked my family to go so I could rest. They brought Brendan to me and laid him in my arms, and we had some time on our own. Then I went to sleep. When I woke up, the sun was shining through the hospital blinds and I couldn't help but think it was the most perfect day.

As soon as I could I asked the nurses to bring Brendan to me. The nurses showed me how to breast-feed him, and just to have him in my arms was magic. Brendan was mine, he belonged to me—what a fantastic feeling.

After we arrived home from the hospital I moved back into the bungalow with Brendan. Every night Mum and Dad helped me bathe him and put him to bed. Dad would take a video of him and they'd hug him and fuss over him. It was a special time.

Brendan was always dressed immaculately. He was like a fragile little china doll. So many people—friends and relatives—kept asking what was going to happen now. Would Jason and I get back together?

I didn't know the answer to that. I knew I still had feelings for Jason but I didn't want to get back together with him just because of Brendan. We were doing fine on our own, my little man and me.

Jason Finally Meets Brendan

Brendan and I were fine in the bungalow—I often lay there at night staring at his beautiful little face, thanking God for bringing this precious joy into my life.

My weight had lessened at that stage. I'd lost fifteen pounds shortly after Brendan's birth, and I was very happy with that. It's strange but I really felt like I had control over my life, and I was determined—if only out of spite—that when Jason saw me I was going to look good. I really took care of myself because I wanted Jason to see me as pretty. And, of course, I was also very aware of the weight I'd put on during my pregnancy.

But the weight didn't stay off for long. Slowly, pound by pound, it piled back on—and when I say piled, it really piled. I had lost fifteen pounds and, gradually over the ensuing months, put thirty back on!

But my weight didn't seem to matter too much to me at that time, I was so proud of being a mum that everything else was irrelevant. There were days when I took Brendan out for a walk, and I couldn't stop smiling at the fact that I was pushing his pram. Going shopping with him was a real treat, and I relished all of the simple things a mother does with a baby like packing his bibs, bottle, diapers and pacifiers into his bag for a day out.

In late September my lawyer phoned with the results of Brendan's DNA test—just as I'd known all along, Jason was the father. There had never been any doubt in my mind, but the news was still overwhelming. Jason had been waiting for this news for more than nine months and I knew that his sleepless nights had finally come to an end.

All day long, I waited for his phone call. Finally, that evening, he called. He told me that he'd gotten the results earlier in the day, but hadn't been able to muster up the courage to call until then.

"I don't know what to say to you," he said. "I don't know if I should start apologizing now and I don't know how the hell I'm ever going to make it up to you. For nine months I thought he wasn't my son and here it is in front of me—he is. And there's no doubt."

I didn't know what to say to him. I felt sorry for him at first. The love I still felt for Jason meant that I couldn't bear to put him through any more angst. Putting aside all of the negative thoughts I had, I arranged to meet him at our house that Sunday. Brendan was just nine weeks old, and I couldn't wait for Jason to finally meet him.

When the Sunday arrived, I dressed Brendan in his best outfit. He looked absolutely gorgeous. Then I started to get ready myself, making an extra effort to look nice. Even though I was heavy, I felt confident. I was the one in control. I wasn't going to get back together with Jason because of Brendan, because I knew I was strong enough to raise Brendan on my own. If Jason and I were going to get back together again, it would be because we still loved each other as much as we had on that day we were married years before. The test for me would be to see whether I could finally forgive and forget. My emotions were all over the place; I didn't know where to turn.

When Jason opened the door he was clearly nervous—and so was I. My legs were like jelly. I took Brendan's carrier to the kitchen table and said to Jason, "Meet our son."

Jason grabbed his tiny little hand and told him he was his daddy. My heart melted. Jason picked him up and held him; he was overcome with emotion, sobbing. I let father and son have their time alone, and when I returned to the house twenty minutes later Jason was still holding Brendan, talking to him.

Just before I left, I went to the back room—the same room I'd always dreamed of turning into a nursery for our children—to change Brendan's diaper. Jason kneeled down on the floor to watch me change Brendan, and was rubbing his soft tummy and his toes. He turned to me and said, "Karen, this is a miracle. Brendan is our little miracle." And I knew exactly what he meant.

> *He turned to me and said, "Karen, this is a miracle. Brendan is our little miracle." And I knew exactly what he meant.*

Endings...and New Beginnings

We agreed to meet the following Sunday, but before the day rolled around we got the news that we'd sold the house. I met Jason at the real-estate agent's office to sign the papers. Jason asked me how Brendan and I were, and asked me to give Brendan a kiss for him. Our conversations were getting calmer and calmer. Gradually we were starting to communicate like a couple again. When I got back to my parents' house, I absolutely broke down. We'd lost our home. My father comforted me, reminding me that it was just a material thing and to keep thanking God I had Brendan—material things come and go. And I knew he was right.

Jason and I continued to meet once a week, but now at my parents' house. Eventually, I had gained almost triple the amount of weight I'd lost after Brendan's birth. I couldn't wear any of the pretty dresses that average-sized women wear, and eventually I got used to wearing tracksuit pants and baggy T-shirts. I was dressing to be comfortable.

Then, out of the blue, Jason asked me if he could come around one night during the week to see Brendan. This was a good opportunity for us to make up lost ground, so I cooked Jason his favorite meal, and I made the excuse that I hadn't had time to eat before he arrived so we could eat together.

Brendan was bathed and in his pajamas ready for Jason. After they'd played together for a little while I was ready to put him to bed. That night Jason stayed and ate with me—normally he would leave straight after seeing Brendan, so I knew that this time he was here to see me, too. We talked for hours; it was magical.

Neither of us dared to mention our split—we didn't want to cause an argument. He looked so handsome and I felt myself open up to him more and more. That night proved to me I still had strong feelings for him.

Before he left, Jason went into Brendan's room and gave him a kiss good-night. I grabbed Jason's hand and told him I wished things were different between us—he said he did, too.

A few visits later, Jason took me by the arms. I really thought he was going to kiss me, but he looked down and said, "I want to thank you from the bottom of my heart for giving me a son. I will never forget what you've done and what you've been through."

No matter how much I tried to lose weight, I had binges to comfort myself. I would eat anything in sight and then feel depressed and ashamed for hours.

I froze, I didn't know what to say. That visit was a breakthrough for us. We agreed on all of the visitations; we were even thinking years ahead about Brendan's future.

Brendan's christening was coming up and I'd planned to have a party at our house with my parents. It was posing some dilemmas for me. I really wanted Jason to be at the church, as he was Brendan's father that was certainly appropriate, but decisions about the rest of the day were proving stressful.

No matter how much I tried to lose weight and look good for the day, I had binges of eating to comfort myself. I would eat anything in sight and then feel depressed and ashamed for hours.

I had binged a lot during our separation and my pregnancy—apart from the baby it was the only way I could make myself happy. I'd eat when I was upset, I'd eat when I was depressed, I'd eat for almost any reason, but it only made me feel ten times worse—so I'd then eat again.

Jason's role in the christening was causing me a lot of grief. I told him he could come to the party, but that there would be people and family members present he wouldn't want to see. I chose my brother and my sister as godparents, and Jason wanted his brother Anthony and his sister-in-law Yolanda to be godparents. That was fine, but I laid it on the line that I didn't want a lot of communication with his family, because we were intending to divorce and it would only complicate things further.

Brendan's christening was a really big deal for Jason and me. We both have quite strong religious backgrounds and our parish priest had been a longtime friend of Jason's. Brendan's christening gown was the same one my brother and sister and I had worn and I was looking forward to Brendan following in that tradition. Instead of losing weight throughout all these preparations, the pounds started to pack on again. I got so excited I would just eat and not care.

On the day of the christening I felt good and I thought I looked pretty good. I think a lot of that was knowing I was going to be spending the whole day with Jason. His car pulled up as I was putting the finishing touches on my makeup and I watched him take a big deep breath—I was doing the same thing. I knew at that moment that I still loved Jason. All the previous night I had been thinking about us spending the day together as a family. Our divorce was due to be finalized in a matter of weeks, yet our communication was improving day by day.

It was a very emotional day for us. Tears began pouring down my face as the priest sprinkled the holy water on Brendan's head. I was overcome with emotion, saddened by the situation that Jason and I were in.

I'd been very nervous about the family photos and had wondered whether Jason was going to be a part of them. I was still a little apprehensive when the time came for them to be taken but our families encouraged us to have pictures together. As Jason and I stood at the altar holding Brendan, our shoulders touched.

I felt as if a surge of electricity had gone through me. We were standing with our son at the same altar where we'd exchanged our marriage vows. I wept again and I could see Jason wiping away tears, too.

I knew Jason still loved me.

That night I ate and ate and ate because I was so happy—bizarre, isn't it? The last thing on my mind at that time was my weight! Some family members took the liberty of telling me how much better I'd look if I lost weight—*thanks very much!* Comments like these only spurred me on to keep eating.

The christening party was a real family celebration. We had the same caterers that Jason and I had had for our wedding, and the christening cake was the top layer of our wedding cake, re-iced. It was a special day. We had balloons, champagne, people cheering, dancing, clapping—a perfect party.

Until it came time for the speeches. Jason came and stood beside me, which made me very nervous. I really wasn't sure if it was right for him to be there. I began by thanking everyone for coming, thanking my parents for all their hard work and thanking God for giving me Brendan. I was relieved when I finished. But then Jason spoke.

He thanked me for giving him the one thing he'd always wanted, and in front of all of my relatives he apologized for making me go through the pregnancy on my own. I was overwhelmed—it was a lovely gesture—but then he turned to me and said, "Karen, you are still my wife and I want to thank you from the bottom of my heart."

Our guests broke into applause but my heart was pounding. He leaned over in front of everyone to kiss me and that was it—I put Brendan into his arms and ran inside the house, away from everyone. In Mum's bedroom I was wracked by tears because I felt completely overwhelmed and confused. All my emotions had been on display—in front of seventy people.

I thought Mum might follow me, but when someone knocked on the door it wasn't her, it was Jason. He slid the door open and found me sobbing my heart out. I could hardly breathe, I was so overcome. He sat down next to me and I demanded to know why he'd done what he did.

He cupped my face in his hands and kissed me, a really passionate kiss. I knew then we would get back together. He told me that he still loved me and I told him I felt the same, and we spent the next twenty minutes talking. We forgot all about the party. We tried to put together all the pieces of the puzzle about why we'd split. I still didn't want to get back together just for Brendan's sake, and neither did he. We made it perfectly clear to each other that it was our love that had reunited us. We both cried with emotion. This horrendous battle was over; we'd come through it.

We made it perfectly clear to each other that it was our love that had reunited us.

As we walked back out to the party, of course all eyes were on us. We announced that we were reconciled and were going to give our marriage another go. Well, everybody was in tears, clapping and cheering. My parents were the last to come up to us. They were overwhelmed with relief and happiness.

I couldn't wait for everyone to leave so I could spend time alone with Jason and Brendan. We talked all night, getting our lives back together, and I knew we would be together forever. We decided we would go back to our priest and tell him, and renew our vows. After all of our time apart, everything fit back together perfectly; there was no doubt Jason and I were meant to be together. It was almost as if we'd woken up from a bad dream.

The very next day, the divorce papers were delivered to our door. As soon as Jason got hold of them, he grabbed some scissors and cut the papers into millions of pieces. We couldn't believe how close we had come to our marriage officially being over!

"I felt exhausted with life."

Laura

Starting Weight: **270** pounds

Current Weight: **154** pounds

116 POUNDS LOST!

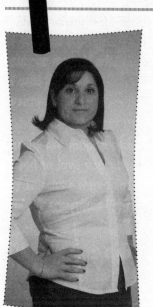

My cousin's wedding day was my lowest point. She'd asked me to be her maid of honor and I was determined to make her wedding day really special. But every minute of that day is vivid in my mind for all the wrong reasons.

I weighed 270 pounds and I hated myself so much. I was disgusted that I couldn't even lose weight for the biggest day in my cousin's life. I'd set myself a target months before, and this day was going to be the day I unveiled my new look in front of family and friends, but I'd failed again. I spent most of the wedding day sobbing.

Surprisingly, even after all of that anguish, I really wasn't ready to change my life. The crunch came a few weeks after the wedding. I was home reading a magazine and I came across the story of a woman who'd had a stroke. She was only thirty when it happened and she'd been fit and healthy all of her life. Next to the story was a box detailing the symptoms she had suffered in the lead-up to the stroke, I felt like I was reading about my own life: high blood pressure, shortness of breath, heart palpitations, anxiety. The list of symptoms was long and I had every one of them!

That's when I started to really panic. For the first time I knew that if I didn't do something about my weight, somebody else would be reading about me. Throughout my life I have lost weight and gained it; it's been a roller-coaster ride for me. But by the time I was twenty-nine, I'd had enough of the diet roller coaster. I felt empty inside and exhausted with life. It was around that time that Karen came into my life. I read an article about her and attended one of her support groups.

She had such an impact on me, but initially I still didn't believe I could do what she's done. I looked at her with such awe—she was amazing—but I thought to myself, *Wow, I'll never be able to achieve what she's achieved.*

Karen really struck a chord with me because she had been so big before and she'd done it herself. And look at her now. She inspired me and helped me rebuild my life from the bottom up.

She helped me learn to believe in myself and it worked. I feel amazing, my life has totally turned upside down. I look back at the pictures of me, and I feel sad to think that my life could've been different if only I'd met someone like Karen sooner. Now I don't waste a minute—there's too much life to live!

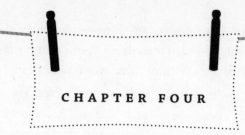

CHAPTER FOUR

Eating for Two

I WAS ECSTATIC THAT JASON AND I WERE BACK TOGETHER.
Along with my happiness came the pounds. I was mounding the weight on.
I was so content—but the happier I got, the bigger
I became. My weight went up and I was feeling
sick. We went to Portarlington for a few days to
get away and I just got sicker and sicker. So I went
to the local doctor—only to discover I was four
weeks pregnant!

> *I had no control over food at all and my weight was ballooning.*

I was thrilled at the thought of another child. Although Brendan was still
very young and having two babies close together was a bit frightening for me,
I would never complain. I'd wanted children for so long.

Losing Control

This pregnancy was the worst time for my weight. I had no control over food
at all and my weight was ballooning. Yet again, I made the excuse that I was
eating for two. Every week I gained more weight. I got to the stage where I just
couldn't, and wouldn't, go out. I had no clothes that would fit me. I had to wear
Jason's tracksuit pants and shirts to feel comfortable.

We'd eat dinner—a big plate of anything—then we'd order pizza and have a family bar of chocolate—all in one sitting. It was nothing for me to have two liters of soda a day, packets of chips; whatever I could fit in, I did.

Brendan was crawling, almost walking, and he was constantly on the go. I was so big I couldn't bend over to pick him up. I had thought I was big when I was pregnant with Brendan but I was much, much bigger this time. I was eight months pregnant when my blood pressure soared and I began to have problems with fluid retention. My ankles were swollen to almost twice their usual size. My doctor warned me many times to eat less, but it went in one ear and out the other. The medical staff even had trouble doing my ultrasounds because there was too much fat on me for the equipment to be effective.

I got to the stage where I just couldn't, and wouldn't, go out.

I figured that once the baby was born, all of the weight would go.

In the meantime I struggled to get in and out of the bathroom, I couldn't hang clothes on the line, and I was too big even to cook food, so we'd end up ordering takeout.

When I was eight months pregnant I was wearing size 26 tops—and they were tight. Trying to sleep was virtually impossible. I could not get comfortable at all. Some nights Jason would sleep on the floor because I needed the whole queen-size bed.

I wouldn't even let Jason see me naked because I was so disgusted at the way I looked.

I got out of breath very easily and our sex life died when I was six months into the pregnancy. I wouldn't even let Jason see me naked because I was so disgusted at the way I looked. A pregnant woman's body is a beautiful thing, but when you are covered in fat, it's not that beautiful, let me tell you. In fact, I was so fat you couldn't actually tell I was pregnant.

Still, when I was hungry I wouldn't think twice about eating, and I'd go to the fridge and pull out cheese, leftover takout, old pizza, all of it. If we didn't have much in the fridge, I'd eat five or six pieces of toast. We always had unsliced bread so we could cut it much thicker and get more butter on it. The bread would be soaked all the way through with butter and jam, and we went through tubs of butter like there was no tomorrow.

If there was nothing at home to eat, I'd make Jason go to the shop and buy more food. It didn't matter what time of day or night it was—I made him go, and he wasn't game to challenge me. I drove Jason crazy. I would eat a king-size block of chocolate like I hadn't seen chocolate for years.

I was so fat you couldn't actually tell I was pregnant.

Jason often blames himself and says he should have drawn my attention to how big I was getting, but it wasn't his fault. Every day was the same; I spent it eating as much as I could. If we went out for dinner, we went to all-you-can-eat restaurants, and literally I ate all that I could! It was nothing for me to empty four or five plates of food in one sitting.

It was always in the back of my mind how big I was. If I was in the shower and Jason walked in, I would demand he get out. I didn't want him in there with me, because I was embarrassed about my body.

And I was big. I took up almost the whole space in the shower cubicle—if I dropped the soap I had no hope of getting down to the floor to pick it up. Jason had to shave my legs for me because I couldn't bend down.

My doctor warned me many times to stop eating so much because my blood pressure was sky-high. In fact, on a weekly basis he warned me that I was eating all of the wrong things but I argued that I needed nourishment for the baby.

Looking back, I can't believe I argued with a doctor!

He told me that he couldn't understand how I was even walking around with such high blood pressure. Not only that, the weight of my ever-expanding tummy and chest put so much pressure on my lungs I was struggling to breathe. Even then, I still didn't really take it seriously. Aside from my weight, everything was perfect. I took it for granted that being a big pregnant woman was just part of life, and I always reasoned that I would lose the weight when I gave birth. Still I was embarrassed about my size with or without clothes.

Every day was the same; I spent it eating as much as I could.

I felt sorry for Jason, too, but this time I wasn't going to tell him he deserved better. Maybe that's why I had no control over my weight—because I knew he loved me no matter what size I was. Another factor in the equation was Brendan, who by the age of one was a real handful. He caused me a lot of stress and again I compensated by eating food such as french fries and pies.

During my checkup at the doctor's, I was weighed. I hated it! My final clinic visit was on my twenty-fifth birthday and I weighed 300 pounds. The first thing the doctor did was check my blood pressure and it was way over what it should have been.

A Difficult Labor

With Brendan I'd had a twenty-two-hour labor and I didn't want the same thing with this baby. The very next day I started to feel pain in my stomach and my chest. As soon as Jason came home he took me straight to the hospital. They put me in the delivery room within half an hour.

My final clinic visit was on my twenty-fifth birthday and I weighed 300 pounds.

Hours ticked by but nothing was happening and I was having visions of this labor taking days. After eight hours of labor I demanded to have a cesarean because I didn't think I could go through hours of pain all over again.

The medical staff got me ready for an epidural. The first one went in and I could feel the coldness running down my spine, but it took another six to make it effective. I had seven epidurals. They simply couldn't get through the fat. I screamed out loud; I just couldn't bear any more pain. It was all because of my weight!

I couldn't breathe and I yelled at Jason to help me. The doctor explained that I couldn't feel myself breathe because I'd had so much anesthetic. So many thoughts were going through my mind—I kept having flashbacks of all our traumas and I constantly compared this birth with Brendan's. But in the back of my mind I always knew it was my fault that I was in so much pain. It was all because of my weight. It was only at that stage, when I was in sheer agony, that I had real regrets about not having tried harder to lose weight. I felt I deserved the pain, and I wanted to end it all. I hoped God would come down and take me.

I had seven epidurals. They simply couldn't get through the fat.

Within minutes, they'd pulled Ryan Ashley Gatt out and the doctor held him up for us to see. He was tiny. He was a beautiful little face staring at us, so much smaller than Brendan.

Jason was over the moon. He'd longed for this experience and had been shattered that he'd missed out on Brendan's birth. The doctors wrapped Ryan up and Jason held him; he wouldn't let him go.

My labor had been hideous, but I now had two sons and I was so very proud and happy. Those two little boys signaled the start of a whole new world for Jason and me. We felt all of our troubles were behind us and we were beginning our life together all over again.

Everything Was Perfect, Except for My Weight

My boys and Jason were the center of my world. I was so proud that I finally had a family of my own. But soon after Ryan was born my weight crept up and up again, and I began to feel quite depressed.

Jason had been trying to tell me politely that I was getting large. He was always encouraging me to lose weight. He'd say, "Karen, I think we need to go on a diet, we're putting on weight. Let's shed it together." Despite the best of intentions we generally lasted about a day.

It was incredible to think that after all the years of not being able to have babies, I now had two under two years old—and what a handful they were. Brendan was thirteen months old when Ryan was born and he was a bundle of energy.

With a new addition to the family, the bungalow just became too small for the four of us. Some nights Brendan would sleep with Mum and Dad so that he wouldn't wake when Ryan screamed for a feeding. But we really needed some space of our own.

There was a house at the corner of my parents' street that had come up for sale and we desperately wanted it. It was perfect as it was so close to Mum and Dad and they were such a huge help to us.

After Christmas and our annual holiday, we moved in. Jason wanted to carry me over the threshold—as if! He nagged me until I agreed, but when he went to lift me I'm sure he almost broke his spine. He couldn't get me off the ground. My family was there, too, so my uncle yelled out, "I'll help." Jason grabbed me from under the arms and my uncle grabbed my feet, and they dragged me through the front door.

I could hear everybody laughing in the background. It was horrible—what a sight I must have been. I laughed at myself, too, on the outside, but in my heart I wanted to die of embarrassment. I seemed to be getting bigger and bigger by the minute. I struggled with my weight so much after Ryan's birth that I was like a balloon ready to pop! If only I had been that simple to deflate, I'd have grabbed the pins myself. Jason and I agreed that our lives were in some ways wasting away because of our weight, but it was no easy matter to shed it. Despite how miserable we were being fat, we didn't change the way we ate.

> *In my heart I wanted to die of embarrassment. I seemed to be getting bigger and bigger by the minute.*

I couldn't stop eating. I always wanted to do something about my weight but I never had the motivation to begin, and always in the back of my mind was the excuse, "Oh well, you're married now, you've got your boys—who cares how you look?" How wrong I was.

I was a true mum. I cooked, cleaned, made bottles, changed diapers, washed clothes and cared for my kids—that was my full-time job and never once did I begrudge anything. Being really content with my life as a wife and mother made me eat! Happy or sad, I ate.

When I had been pregnant I had continually said to myself, "Once I have Ryan I'll do something about it." But once I had Ryan, I didn't. He gave me another excuse not to. How many times did I tell myself, I was too tired, too busy—too anything to lose weight? I always had an excuse.

> *I couldn't stop eating. Happy or sad, I ate.*

While we were on our summer vacation it was too hot to cook, so that was my excuse for eating takeout. Each night we'd take the kids down to the beach and eat pizza or fish and chips for dinner, followed up by a double scoop of ice cream. We'd then go back to the trailer and watch TV while polishing off nuts, popcorn and handfuls of candy washed down with two liters of soda before we rolled into bed. This routine went on for the three weeks we were away.

Quite often the kids and Jason would go for a swim, but there was no way I was going for a dip! I'd sit by the beach watching them—sweating underneath my long shirt and shorts—and I could hear Brendan calling out to me to go into the water. "Mum, Mum, Mum." It broke my heart to hear him, but I just couldn't do it.

I truly was a beached whale. When I look now at the family videos I cringe—the Grand Canyon was small in comparison with my bum! I went to the beach wrapped up in the biggest clothes I could find and a blanketlike towel.

As alcohol, smoking and drugs are addictions for other people, food was one for me. I was an addict and there seemed to be nothing that could break the spell food had over me.

I hated my weight and I always desperately wanted to do something about it, but I didn't have the motivation. As alcohol, smoking and drugs are addictions for other people, food was one for me. I was an addict and there seemed to be nothing that could break the spell food had over me.

There were times when Brendan, thinking I was still pregnant, would grab my tummy and say "Ryan?" I'd have to explain to him that Mummy wasn't having a baby, she was just fat. That nearly broke my heart. If such a young child could see so clearly how big I was, I could only imagine what other people thought.

As the kids began to grow and become more active, naturally they wanted to do more active things like going to the park. Brendan would ask me to go and I'd say yes, but even though it was just around the corner from our house I had to drive there because I couldn't manage the walk. My parents lived four houses away from us and walking there felt like a two-mile hike to me. I missed out on so much fun with my boys because I just couldn't manage it physically. And often when they'd have a nap in the afternoon, so would I because I was exhausted.

I lived my life thinking "If only I were slim" and "I'll start my diet on Monday."

I lived my life thinking "If only I were slim" and "I'll start my diet on Monday." Familiar?

I hated being seen naked—absolutely hated it—and I hated Jason touching my stomach. My stomach was hanging down so much I couldn't see my toes—or anything else. Naturally, my weight affected our sex life, too.

When I was at my heaviest, I found a part-time job working in a kitchen at a reception center. I had to buy a uniform and I couldn't find one bigger than size 26. I had to have one specially made in a size 32, and in the end I only lasted three months in the job because I was so embarrassed about my size.

Food continued to be a real obsession for me. If I had a chocolate bar in the pantry or some cookies or cake, I couldn't just leave them there. I would eat the whole package. If the kids opened a packet of chocolate cookies and had one each, the fact the cookies were there would eat away at me all day until I went into the pantry and scarfed down the whole package. I wouldn't rest until they were all gone. This will sound bizarre, but I was actually haunted by food—voices in my mind would say, "Karen, there's cake in the cupboard—eat it, eat it." And literally the voices would not go away until I had eaten the whole cake.

I was actually haunted by food—voices in my mind would say, "Karen, there's cake in the cupboard—eat it, eat it." And the voices would not go away until I had eaten the whole cake.

No matter how much I tried to ignore those thoughts, I couldn't get rid of them until I got up and polished off the cake or cookies—then I was fine and would be back to normal. Obesity is a disease, and it's a mental disease as much as a physical one.

My whole body was deteriorating before my eyes. My periods stopped, my blood pressure was near the boiling point and I could hear my own heart absolutely pounding, trying to keep up with me. My feet were always swollen and I would sweat as if I'd just run a marathon even when doing nothing. As soon as I finished my shower I would be dripping with sweat again. Jason put a ceiling fan in the bedroom for me, but it didn't make much difference.

The kids had a little inflatable pool in the backyard and on hot summer days, we'd fill it up so they could keep cool. Often Jason would go out and sit in the pool with them and encourage me to come out, too. When I got in, though, everybody else would have to get out to make room for me and, sure enough, as soon as I sat down the water would rise up over the edge of the pool and overflow into the yard. Brendan would laugh at me and yell, "Look. Mummy—Mummy too fat!"

I could see my kids and Jason spending quality time together and I couldn't join in. But Jason was wonderful, he always had words of comfort for me. Whenever I was feeling down about my weight, he'd say, "Karen, I love you as much as the day I met you, I don't care about your weight."

Every Monday I'd say to myself, "Today I'll start my diet." The morning would go well, I'd be very careful about what I ate, but I never did any exercise. I'd manage to make it through to the afternoon but usually by dinner I'd start to pick at food, and that would be it—the diet would be over until the next Monday came along. Four days was the longest stretch I could manage on any diet; I'd lose two pounds during the four days, and put on two and a half a week later!

Four days was the longest stretch I could manage on any diet; I'd lose two pounds during the four days, and put on two and a half a week later.

I was terrified of food—it had control over me.

I'd go to the cupboard and the cookies would be open and I'd think to myself, *One cookie won't hurt,* then the next hour I'd go back again. *Just one more...* By the end of the day the package was gone—and so was the diet!

I think I repeated that sort of diet for at least eight months. But not one day went by without me thinking about my weight. It got to the stage where I was terrified of food because it had control over me. I couldn't stop myself eating and the more people told me I had to lose weight, the more I ate. It was as if an inner voice was saying, "Don't worry, Karen, eat more."

But the terror wasn't enough to push that one button that would prompt me to do something about it. Until Mother's Day 1999. The morning after the Mother's Day dance was the biggest turning point in my life. It was the dawning of a whole new world. For some reason from the moment I woke up something in my heart had changed and I knew it was truly the beginning of my new life.

From the moment I woke up something in my heart had changed and I knew it was truly the beginning of my life.

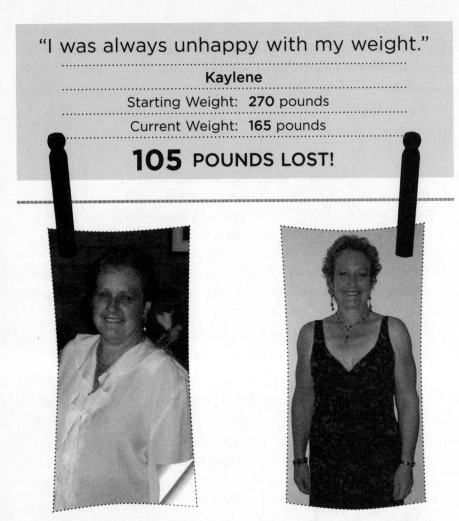

"I was always unhappy with my weight."

Kaylene

Starting Weight: **270** pounds

Current Weight: **165** pounds

105 POUNDS LOST!

I was always unhappy with my weight. I had tried lots and lots of different diets with varied success, but the weight always crept back on. For years I had yo-yoed up and down and I had a wide collection of clothes of different sizes in my wardrobe.

I'd always hated photos of myself, but when I saw a photo of myself from my parents' fiftieth wedding anniversary party, I knew I couldn't hide my weight problem anymore. I felt uncomfortable in my clothes, I had problems with my feet and my hips ached.

My sister-in-law told me about Karen's support group and said she was going, so I jumped at the chance and said I would go, too. Karen changed my life. She inspired me to put in the effort to lose weight. I could see that Karen had been able to lose her weight, so I thought if she could do it, so could I. I found that the support sessions, which included walking and being weighed in, helped keep me on track. I think the combination of walking and the sweat sessions helped burn off the pounds. As time went on, I discovered that I enjoyed the exercise more than I ever had before. I found myself doing all sorts of other activities as well, like going to the gym, cycling, swimming and walking.

When I met Karen I was a single mother of two children. My husband had died sixteen years before. I had been out with a few men during that time, but had mostly been on my own. I think my weight had hampered my ability to find another partner. As I lost weight, my confidence gradually improved and I started going out with my friends again, hoping that now that I was at a more attractive weight I might be lucky enough to find another partner to share my life with. I met a wonderful man and we fell in love! Thanks to the Clothesline Diet, I have a new life.

CHAPTER FIVE

A New Beginning

THE MORNING AFTER THE MOTHER'S DAY DANCE I MADE MYSELF a coffee but instead of the two teaspoons of sugar I normally stirred through it, I had none. As I sat at the kitchen table I visualized what my new life was going to be like. I could actually see myself doing things I'd never done before. Playing with my boys, dancing with my husband, wearing beautiful clothes.

I visualized what my new life was going to be like.

The biggest hurdle, naturally, was working out how I was going to lose the weight. I sat and thought really long and hard about achieving my dream.

Something was different this time; I just knew that I didn't want my old life anymore.

The very idea of going yet again to a weight-loss center or starving myself on crash diets as I'd done as a teenager sent shivers down my spine. I couldn't go back to any of those programs because they hadn't worked for me in the past, and I had no faith that this time would be any different. I also quietly made a promise to myself not to tell anyone, except Jason, what I was doing because I didn't want to be seen as a failure yet again if I didn't achieve my goal.

Something was different this time; I just knew that I didn't want my old life anymore. I started to have quite positive thoughts. I told myself that I deserved to be happy. I deserved to live a normal life, and I deserved to do something for myself.

Creating the Clothesline Diet

Formulating a diet plan was almost like solving a puzzle. I had to start from square one and work out each step that would take me to my goal. I resolved to myself that if I was really going to do this, I had to start right there and then, not the next day or the day after that. So I got up and grabbed the trash can and went straight to the fridge.

Cleaning the Cupboards

The first important step was getting rid of all of the food I thought was fatty—and there was a lot there! I would have to rebuild every piece of my day-to-day life, and my fridge and the food in it had become a key part of my world, so that was the place to start.

Butter and margarine had question marks over them because I wasn't sure what I could replace them with, so for now they stayed. But all the jellies, honey, peanut butter and cream-cheese spreads went straight into the trash. From now on, anything that was going to go on our bread or muffins would have to be low-fat. I knew that I could buy fat-free muffins, and I wanted to replace our white bread with something a little healthier, too.

The whole milk went into the bin to be replaced by fat-free milk. Then we got to the cheeses—and believe me, I loved cheese! When I sat and really looked I couldn't believe how much cheese we had in our fridge. Soft cheese, cream cheese, Swiss cheese, cheddar cheese, sliced cheese—out they all went.

The next step was the soda shelf. Yes, I had a whole shelf of different sorts of soda! There was no doubt this move would lead to something of a backlash from Jason and the kids, but that was too bad. I knew it all had to go. I threw every bottle of soda in the bin and replaced them with a jug of water.

The fridge and I were healthier already.

The pantry was next. My pantry was an obese person's paradise! Didn't we love cookies and crackers—oh boy, we had all sorts of junk food to choose from. We also had peanuts and all the snack food you could imagine. We had enough snack food to feed a small country.

I knew it would be too much for me just to cut out all the food I had been used to eating all my life, so I looked for alternatives. Rather than giving up the foods I loved, I replaced the "bad" foods with

This plan wasn't like a traditional diet at all.

healthier versions. I never looked at what I was doing as a diet in the usual sense, which can conjure up negative images of starvation and punishment. This plan wasn't like a traditional diet at all. Instead I wanted to change my lifestyle without having to sacrifice my favorite meals. And most of all, I didn't want to spend my time cooking one meal for me, one for Jason and another for the kids.

I discovered ways to make the food that we enjoyed as a family healthy to eat. There are so many low-fat and low-sugar foods on the market; they aren't that hard to find. We would still have muffins and baked goods, but they would be low-fat and low-sugar brands. And the harshest critics—my children—would not be able to taste the difference. And potato chips—we had so many flavors of potato chips. They all went in the trash, and I would replace them with healthy alternatives such as rice crackers.

It is pointless totally depriving yourself of everything you love. Losing weight doesn't need to be a torturous process.

It is pointless totally depriving yourself of everything you love. Losing weight doesn't need to be a torturous process. All of these changes are simple lifestyle changes, and honestly my family didn't even notice the difference, aside from all of us feeling so much healthier.

Clearing out our cupboards was a cleansing step for me; it showed me that I was serious about my health. I felt I'd taken huge steps forward just by getting rid of all the food that was bad for us.

Stocking a Low-Fat Kitchen

The next step was to go to the supermarket and replace everything.

I made our beds, had my shower and off I went. Like a woman possessed, I had a very clear mission that day. I spent hours in the supermarket. I looked at every food product in every aisle, from the top shelf to the bottom. I read every label and studied the products thoroughly. I was soaking up information that was going to change my and my family's lives. I had an idea of what was healthy and what was unhealthy and I used my intuition as a guide in looking for low-sugar, low-fat, high-fiber and whole-grain foods.

Thinking about Jason and the boys was a big incentive for me, too. This wasn't something I was just doing for myself. I was doing this for my children and my husband, as well. And it made it so much easier for me, too, to be eating the same food as them. I can't count the number of diets I'd tried that involved special food for me, while everybody else ate other meals. Cooking two or three sets of food for every meal just didn't appeal to me, and I know it is a huge stumbling block for others—who has the time? That's when dieting becomes too hard and you give up.

I got on the scales that night and weighed in at 283 pounds. I had a very long road ahead of me.

You have to work at everything to achieve your goals and losing weight is no different, but there are ways of making it much easier. While I was searching the supermarket I came across a light cream-cheese spread, which was my answer to margarine and butter. Perfect. I wanted to replace the starchy white bread I had always bought before with something healthier, so I added whole-grain bread to the cart.

I knew, too, that the kids would have major objections to the water jug so I looked at fruit juices with no added sugar and bought some healthy replacements for the soda we would no longer have. I was sure to stock up on a variety of healthy fruits and vegetables, too, for salads, side dishes and fruit salads.

With my cart loaded up with new food, my mission was accomplished.

When Jason came home from work that afternoon and went to the fridge, the first thing he noticed was the water jug standing where the soda used to be.

He looked at me, startled, and said, "What's going on here?" I told him that this was it—I was changing my life. When he opened the pantry, he got shock number two. We had all sorts of different cereals that were high in fiber and low in fat and sugar—no more chocolate or sugar-coated cereals. When he saw the fat-free milk in the fridge, he said, "Oh my God, Karen—how are we supposed to get used to this?" But I knew we would. We were going to make this work.

I got on the scales that night and weighed in at 283 pounds. I knew I had a very long road ahead of me.

Committing to Change

When we woke the following morning, out came the high-fiber, low-fat cereal and the fat-free milk. It felt strange to watch Jason and the boys eating mountains of toast smothered with butter and jam without joining them, but I was determined. My willpower was extraordinarily strong. I was excited, but realistically I didn't know how long I could stick it out. It was a real test; my mind and my body were challenging one another.

Each day gave me another confidence boost.

After the first few days of sticking to the plan, I felt really good. Each day gave me another confidence boost.

At that stage, I thought that I should probably talk to my doctor, too. He gave me an invaluable tip—to go and buy myself a bowl, such as a noodle bowl or soup bowl, and eat every meal from that bowl. He had also told me never to overrun the bowl, and not to pile it high. He said I should replace my plate with the bowl to get myself in a routine.

I picked out a bowl, and that was what I used for breakfast, lunch and dinner. Everything that went over the edge of the bowl was food I didn't need.

Because I'd had high blood pressure, he also wanted to monitor my blood pressure closely. We agreed on a time once a week when I would go to him to be weighed. Knowing that I had that meeting with him was another real incentive for me to stick to the diet.

Walking the Clothesline

The hardest part was, literally, trying to walk.

I knew that I wasn't going to lose weight unless I did some form of exercise. Walking was the most realistic option, but I was a very big girl and had difficulty doing so. I was so embarrassed by the thought of walking down the street, I decided to walk around my backyard. I just wasn't ready to face the world and I couldn't bear the thought of people seeing me waddling around the street. In any case, I had trouble squeezing out the front door.

My backyard was tiny. It was a little concrete courtyard with a clothesline in the middle, but I didn't let that bother me. I wasn't going to push myself too hard; I just wanted to take a few steps and see how it went.

I could only do five minutes before my lungs started to constrict and

I thought I was going to have a heart attack. When I reached that point I stopped, but I was still very pleased with myself—I'd walked for five minutes. I can't tell you how much of an achievement that was for me.

Mind you, those first five minutes of walking felt like an hour. But I had done what I'd set out to do and I had such a sense of pride. I had overcome a huge mental hurdle.

That first day I walked in circles around our clothesline and I counted down every minute. By the time I finished I was covered in sweat and puffing like a steam train. The kids were watching me through the kitchen window and I could see the looks on their faces. I'm sure they thought Mum was losing her mind. They couldn't understand what I was doing.

Each day when I finished my walk I felt better than the day before. The mental hurdles were coming down step by step.

The next day came and I said to myself, "Yesterday I did five minutes; today I will do six." And I did. I didn't worry about how fast or slow I walked; it wasn't about speed, it was just about putting one foot in front of the other. Each day when I finished my walk I felt better than the day before. The mental hurdles were coming down step by step.

The weekly appointments with my doctor became crucial because he reinforced my achievement. I was losing two and half pounds each week and he was extremely proud of me. I was proud of me, too. Knowing I was going to be weighed when I saw him really inspired me, and once I began to lose weight and could see results, the whole program became so much easier. Seeing the rewards of my work on the scales motivated me even more.

I was losing two and half pounds each week.

Living the Clothesline Diet

I was careful to never set unrealistic goals. I just did what I could. Each day I thought of new ways of changing my diet. I started to drink two or three glasses of water before I ate my lunch and dinner. It was an effort, but it made me feel quite full before I sat down to eat. I tried to drink eight glasses of water a day. It was hard initially because I was so used to drinking sugary soft drinks. In comparison, the taste of water was bland. The easiest way for me to adjust was just to have a sip here and there. It took me about six weeks to like drinking water, and now I can't live without it.

For breakfast I'd have high-fiber cereal and low-fat milk with a cup of tea, or I'd have a slice of whole-grain toast with low-fat cream cheese spread. And I was really happy with that. This helped start my day off right with plenty of energy and kept me satisfied all morning.

Sugar had always been a problem for me. I drank a lot of coffee with two or three teaspoons of sugar in it. I knew my diet wouldn't work if I just stopped cold turkey. So I cut everything down gradually. I would have a little less sugar every day, until I was having none. I haven't had sugar in my tea or coffee for three years now.

It would have been pointless to cut out too much too quickly; that would be a quick recipe for failure. Cutting down on the bad foods and replacing them gradually made it so I didn't even notice the difference.

During winter I really loved having soup for lunch, and the low-fat instant soups were great. There are so many different flavors available I never got bored with them. In summer I'd make up big bowls of fresh fruit salad and I ate as much fruit as I wanted. My afternoon snacks were low-fat yogurt or a granola bar or more fruit.

Dinner was more of a challenge and it took me a little while to transform our regular meals from high-fat to low-fat. We experimented a lot!

The skin from roast chicken used to be my favorite food, but that had to go. I started taking all the fat and skin off chicken. You can cook chicken so many ways, but my favorite way of cooking it became boiling it. I put the steamer on, placed the chicken on the bottom with a whole lot of different vegetables on top and I cooked them all together.

I would also boil some eggs, and make a little egg and low-fat mayonnaise salad for us to have with our chicken and vegetables. This was something novel for us because our chicken had always been fried or roasted in loads of fat, but the kids and Jason all loved that dinner. It became a family favorite.

Whenever I was cooking meat, I replaced the cooking fat or oil with water. I'd just drizzle some water over the pan and that's how I fried. We loved mashed potatoes, so instead of mashing them with full-cream milk and butter, I'd use skim milk and a little light cream cheese. It's delicious.

We had a lot of fish and salad. I'd grill some fish, and have loads of salad and steamed vegetables. These were such simple meals that we all enjoyed, and after a little while we really didn't miss the taste of fatty, stodgy, fried food. I made big pots of minestrone soup, piled high with vegetables. There is no fat in that soup at all and the kids totally demolish it. They love it.

I never followed any calorie counters or plans—I didn't have the time! I'm not a doctor—I'm simply an everyday mum and I was just following basic common sense.

The new plan was easier on the wallet, too. Of course we saved money by not having late-night snacks like pizza and chocolate, but we also saved money because healthy food can be cheaper than junk food. For example, six apples is about equal in price to a packet of cookies, and they last longer.

I never missed a day of walking—not once. If it was raining outside, I'd put my jacket on and walk. I loved going for that walk even if it was just for a few minutes; that was my time and I was proud of every minute I added to my routine. Regardless of what the kids were doing inside—Jason was always home to look after them when I walked, and I could hear them giving him a hard time—that walk was my time.

I never followed any calorie counters or plans. I'm not a doctor. I'm simply an everyday mum following basic common sense.

During my walks I really began to think about doing a few more things for myself. Simple things like taking a few minutes longer in the shower instead of rushing in and out became important to me. I really wanted to care for myself. Every day I set myself a challenge to do something for myself; it might be something as simple as painting my nails or shaving my legs, but it felt good to do things for myself.

When I hit my eighth minute I was still puffing, but I'd lost eighteen pounds by then. My doctor had warned me that the first few pounds I'd lose would come off quite quickly, but still I was extremely proud of myself. Jason told me he was beginning to see a difference in my weight and that really spurred me on, too.

The way my clothes fit was a telltale sign and by the time I'd lost eighteen pounds, I was beginning to notice a difference in my wardrobe. Those size

24 shirts were just a little looser around the buttons. After being obese for so long, the smallest amount of weight loss made a difference.

Now, the food temptations are constantly there—don't get me wrong. Food is in front of you wherever you turn and it's pretty easy to just think *One more cookie won't hurt.* That's when you have to be firm with yourself and be strong. I rewarded myself whenever I resisted temptation. I reminded myself of the goal I wanted to achieve and of what I had already achieved, and that helped me through.

From as far back as I can remember my weight had been a battle, but this time it was one I was winning.

Every time a chocolate bar loomed before me, I'd say to myself, "No, Karen, be proud." And I was. And, you know, it gave me a bigger buzz knowing I had beaten the cravings rather than having the few minutes of pleasure—and hours of guilt—of succumbing.

And there wasn't a day that went by that I didn't ask God for courage to help me through the battle.

I never set out to lose weight for anybody else—I did this totally for myself. I'd suffered in a life of teasing and taunting because of my weight and this was my chance to prove I could rise above it. This was my chance to show all of the doubters what I could do. My chance to show the world that my life was worth something. But I knew it wouldn't come without an effort.

Soon I'd lost 20 pounds, then 30, then 40.

Still, if I could achieve this, it would mean I could do anything I had ever dreamed of.

The Pounds Come Off

Losing weight was the biggest battle of my life—my whole life. From as far back as I can remember my weight had been a battle, but this time it was one I was winning. Each visit to my doctor brought me more and more encouragement. He said to me, "Karen, whatever you're doing—stick to it." Soon I'd lost 20 pounds, then 30, then 40. Jumping on scales had always been such a nightmare for me, but now it showed me that I was winning. My blood pressure began to come down, too.

I gradually increased my speed while I was walking, and I lifted my arms and really pumped them instead of letting them dangle down beside me. I was determined.

It took about three months for me to really get used to my new way of doing things but eventually the changes became a natural part of my life. Cooking became a lot easier because I knew what foods to use in place of the fat-filled ones. When we went out for dinner, I'd ask the staff to grill my fish with lemon juice or not put any dressing on my salad. Little changes that add up to pounds—and it

Eventually the changes became a natural part of my life.

all came naturally. It wasn't a struggle. I had the occasional glass of red wine, but I mainly stuck to water and fresh orange juice. If we went to other people's houses for dinner, I didn't want to be rude and not eat. I also didn't want my weight loss to become an excuse for not going out, and I made the effort to go whenever people asked us over. But I was conscious of what I was eating, so instead of scoffing a big slice of lasagna, I'd eat half or a quarter of what was on my plate, or I'd be sure to eat more healthy side dishes like salads and vegetables.

I learned how to control food and fight my cravings.

I'd have days where I longed for chocolate or candy—who doesn't? But instead of running to the candy jar I dipped the tip of my little finger in the sugar bowl and sucked the tiniest amount of sugar off. Strange as it sounds, it killed my sugar cravings instantly.

I reasoned with myself that fruit was healthy and I could eat as much of it as I wanted. If I felt a little hungry or craved something sweet, I'd go to the huge bowl of fruit salad I kept in my fridge and have as much as I liked.

I picked reward days, too. Every Thursday when Jason went to darts and the kids were in bed, I'd run a bath, give myself a facial and paint my nails. That was my time to do something for myself and feel good. I made a conscious effort to not allow food to control me anymore. I learned how to control food

If I felt depressed, or down, food wasn't my source of comfort anymore.

and fight my cravings. If my mind was telling me to eat, I had to learn how to overcome it. I had to learn how to stop using food as a pick-me-up, too. If I felt depressed, or down, food wasn't my source of comfort anymore.

I used to make excuses for being hungry and I'd search for food out of sheer boredom. I had nothing to do, so I'd eat. I overcame that by enjoying myself, going for another walk or doing something else for me.

I also listened to my heart and not my mind. I used to talk down to myself. I spent so many years telling myself, "You're not worth it...you'll never do this"—all sorts of negative thoughts went through my head. And, of course, when you constantly tell yourself you won't do something, you don't! It was a huge shift for me mentally to say to myself, "I am worth this, my life is worth living. I deserve this." It had to come from my heart, though, not my head.

As I got more and more confidence, I walked laps of my whole backyard, not just around the clothesline. I walked around the edge of our property as I added minute after minute.

I was prepared for my weight loss to slow down—and it did. The first 44 pounds came off quite easily. Then I had to start really getting rid of the fat.

Beating the Plateaus

The first real plateau came about two months into my diet. I was sticking to my plan and walking every day but for three weeks my weight didn't move. I really started to get down about it and I did a lot of crying in those weeks. I started to tell myself, "This is it, I'm never going to get to my goal."

Jason was very supportive and encouraging. He told me not to give up and when I'd open up the fridge to pig out, he was there reminding me of my goals all the time. I'd let it all out and have a good cry and then I'd feel better. When I was standing at the fridge tempted to binge, Jason would say, "Go for another walk." And I did. That's how I got over those negative feelings. That clothesline almost became my best friend!

I also tried to vary my exercise to keep losing weight. I added some sit-ups to my routine each day. I did twenty-five before I went to bed each night. My sit-ups really achieved results; I could feel my stomach changing.

The Ten-Week Cycle

I devised a ten-week plan for myself. I'd really work hard for eight weeks, then maintain my weight for two weeks. So I planned my life in ten-week cycles and it worked. From the first week of the plan I followed the same routine for eight weeks. My meals were varied, but always low- or no-fat. Then for two weeks afterward I would maintain my weight. I still followed the same diet pattern, but if we went out for dinner I'd allow myself a piece of chocolate cake and I'd eat half, sharing with Jason.

During my maintaining period, if the kids wanted a bag of chips I'd eat a couple, or if we were out for a Sunday drive, we'd treat ourselves to the mini ice-cream cones from McDonald's. I'd have maybe half and then give the rest to Jason. I never ate a full one.

I didn't want to constantly diet through to my goal weight, because I was always worried about what would happen after I reached my weight—how would I maintain it? Everybody is faced with temptations and I didn't want to reach the weight I'd worked so hard for and then blow it because I didn't know how to control my eating when I wasn't dieting.

It is really important to have some sort of maintaining period while you are dieting to teach yourself how to eat. Those weeks taught me how much I could eat of certain foods without putting on weight. If I put on weight during my maintaining period I knew the next time it came around I had to alter how much I ate.

By the time I reached my goal weight I knew exactly what and how much I could, and couldn't, eat. I knew that if I wanted to eat cheesecake, I could eat eight spoonfuls before I put on weight. And it has worked! I've maintained my goal weight now for eight years. I rewarded myself during those two weeks for the hard work, but I also wanted to find out how things would be when I reached my goal weight. I allowed myself to eat what I wanted, within reason, then I'd see if I had gained weight. If I hadn't gained any weight I knew I was balancing everything.

And I never starved once. I had three meals a day with snacks in between and I was feeling healthier than ever before. I walked every day—no excuses. I never stopped walking or doing sit-ups during my maintaining period. I never, ever made excuses to avoid my exercise.

Learning How to Eat Again

In order to change my life, I had to disregard all my old habits and start from scratch. Every step I took gave me more confidence to keep going.

Before I started my diet, I never really sat down and enjoyed a meal because I was always rushing around, feeding the kids or getting dinner for Jason. But when I started my plan I made a point of sitting down to eat my meal and enjoying it properly. I chewed everything much more slowly and I savored the taste. Apart from really enjoying the taste of my meal, I actually felt full much more quickly, which meant I ate less and didn't feel bloated for hours. Often I would find that halfway through dinner I was already full.

> *I knew that I was heading in the right direction, and this gave me even more motivation to keep going.*

At night, Jason and I loved to sit down together and watch TV after the kids were in bed. That was our quiet time. It was also the time when we ate snacks. Before I started my diet, it was nothing for us to eat a full family-sized block of chocolate or scoff down chips like there was no tomorrow. Instead of junk food, though, now I'd bring out the fruit salad bowl, and treat it as dessert. I found grapes particularly helpful—I'd put a big plate of grapes on the coffee table and we'd always end up eating a lot of them. I always had my water bottle next to me, too.

What I was doing really wasn't a diet in the traditional sense. I didn't starve myself and I ate everything I wanted—I just replaced foods. It was more of a lifestyle change—I was teaching myself how to eat all over again.

Setting Small Goals—and Staying Motivated

Four months after I changed my eating plan, my high blood pressure had totally disappeared. For the first time in years, my blood pressure was normal. That was such an achievement for me. I really felt good about it—seeing positive changes like that was exciting.

Cleaning out my wardrobe was the best. That day was a real highlight—I got such a buzz from taking my big, fat size 24 and 26 clothes and throwing them out. I was around size 20 at that stage and I was determined those clothes were never, ever coming back into my wardrobe!

I knew that I was heading in the right direction, and this gave me even more motivation to keep going. I'd lost nearly 55 pounds and I was walking for twenty minutes a day. I was on top of the world. When I'd first started walking for just five minutes, it was like being in labor again; I had really felt I couldn't do it. Walking for twenty minutes a day was more than I had ever imagined doing. Jason and my family were so proud of me.

I was nowhere near my goal weight yet. But reaching those targets I'd set along the way kept me going. People were giving me compliments and telling me I was looking great, all of which made me feel like I was really achieving something.

I had days when I did struggle; it wasn't easy, by any means. And I had weeks when my weight plateaued and didn't budge. I was losing on average four and a half pounds a week, but some weeks it wouldn't come off and I'd work a little harder for the next week. The most important thing was that the weight was always going down—not up.

I got to the stage where the backyard just wasn't big enough and I felt ready to head out onto the street. One Monday morning I thought, *Today, instead of the yard, I'm going outside*. I was really nervous about people seeing me. Opening that back gate and walking out was scary. I took my water bottle with me, using it as a weight.

I had a lot of mental hurdles to overcome about walking in public, and when I took those first few steps on the street all I could think about was people staring at me and laughing. But once I'd started, it actually felt good. I kept my goal weight firmly in mind as I walked, and that kept me going.

Some days I sat down and visualized myself walking into a room full of people wearing the most beautiful gown. I'd see myself with my head held high, walking through the crowd while everybody smiled at me, no whispers or sideways stares. It felt good imagining the looks on their faces when they saw me after I'd lost weight.

I set little goals for myself all the time. If I had a function coming up, I'd set a goal weight to achieve by that time. If I had a wedding to go to, I'd weigh myself the day I got the invitation, and then set a target of pounds to lose for the day. That gave me another incentive so I'd work a little harder to reach my goal.

Seven months after starting my diet, we received the invitation for my cousin's wedding in November. There were six weeks before the wedding and having that wedding date in my mind gave me a real incentive to lose more weight. I added a few more minutes to my walk each day and did a few extra sit-ups, and two weeks before the wedding I went out to buy a dress. I bought size 20, but it was a little big. I tried it on again the week before the wedding and it was even bigger, so Mum took it in for me. I was actually a size 18. I couldn't believe it!

The day of the wedding I really started to see just how much my life was turning around. So many people—friends and relatives—came up to me complimenting me on how I looked, and I could see that Jason was really proud. He was showing me off around the room and that felt good. I held my head high that night. I felt on top of the world!

Something to Celebrate

Finally, two weeks after my cousin's wedding, I broke the 220-pound barrier. I stood on the scales and they flicked around before my eyes until they stopped at 220.

Wow, what an amazing feeling!

I'd been over 220 pounds for as long as I could remember. To see the scales at 220 was incredible. That morning my willpower skyrocketed. I couldn't wait to tell Jason, and when I did he was over the moon for me, too. I had worked so hard to get to 220 pounds, and something as simple as that made me feel as though I'd won the lottery. Knowing I'd done it on my own without weight-loss centers and prepackaged food was an even bigger bonus.

Christmas was just six weeks away and I wanted to break the 200-pound barrier for Christmas. That was my gift to myself. It was a big task but I set myself goals along the way and this really helped. That summer (Australian summers start in December) I wanted to buy my first swimsuit. I wanted to be able to go to the beach and chase my kids in the sand and do the things I'd missed out on for so many years. Things I'd longingly watched other mums do. So I had a clear target in my head, and having that goal in my mind made it much easier. I worked especially hard for three months to get my weight down.

At this stage Jason started to notice I was also a much happier person. I was really coming out of my shell and I had much more self-confidence. My paranoia about my weight was subsiding, too.

Christmas posed a dilemma for me, though, because I knew there would be so much food. I counteracted that by planning the two weeks around Christmas and New Year to be my maintaining time. That meant I could taste the food I wanted without breaking my diet and without feeling I was missing out.

I really wanted to have something nice to wear for New Year's Eve, too. Every year we celebrated New Year's Eve at a dinner-dance—we'd been going to the same one for years. But I wanted this one to be special.

While I was shopping a few weeks before Christmas I came across a dress shop that I had never been able to buy anything from before. This time I walked in, and as I flicked through the racks of clothes I found a dress I liked. I took a size 24 and headed for the change room to try it on.

The sales assistant looked at me, puzzled, and said, "Darling, you are not a size 24." I'd had to be reminded that I wasn't that size anymore. I swapped it for a size 20 and went into the change room.

The dress looked pretty good but I rarely wore dresses and my confidence just wasn't there. It was a little loose around my tummy so the assistant swapped it for a size 18. That fit—and it looked good. A size 18. Wow! It was such a thrill to be able to buy clothes with a label that read 18. I knew I was around that size but I was too unsure to ever buy anything with an 18 on it. I always bought bigger, just in case. But that label confirmed my dreams—I was winning the battle.

For the first time in my life, I'd started to control the food; the food wasn't controlling me.

But I was still nowhere near my goal weight, and I wasn't really sure about the dress, so I took Mum and Jason into the shop for their opinion. The look on Jason's face said it all—he was beaming. He told me I looked beautiful and I believed him. Mum was speechless.

So I bought the dress. In the weeks leading up to Christmas I kept really working hard. I didn't quite get down under 200 pounds by Christmas because my weight plateaued again. But I still felt good.

Christmas Eve was once again our night to cook dinner, and we were having everybody over. The dinner I cooked was very healthy and very low in fat. We had grilled fish as an entrée, and the main course was roast chicken and beef with vegetables. I cooked the meat in the oven with water—no oil. For dessert we had fruit salad and low-fat ice cream, and I made banana splits for the kids.

That Christmas went well. It was a really special time for us. Everybody stayed over and ate and ate, but I still had a clear idea in my mind of what I wanted to weigh and what my goal was and I stuck to it. For the first time in my life, I'd started to control the food; the food wasn't controlling me.

With Christmas over, we headed off to the beach for our holidays.

I hadn't quite reached my goal yet so I was still a little unsure about wearing a swimsuit. I wore a one-piece and shorts over the top.

I never felt like I was sacrificing anything.

That was a great time—we walked everywhere. I purposely didn't take my scale with me because I wanted to have a break from it. Every day I wondered how much I weighed, and I contemplated going and buying one, but I managed to get by.

Each night we took the kids for a walk to get an ice cream. They'd get cones piled high and I'd eat a small low-fat cone or a small bowl of fruit salad. We had loved having fish and fries by the water with the kids, and we still did, but instead of having fried fish I'd have a piece of grilled fish with lemon, and fruit salad afterward, and that was delicious.

I never felt like I was sacrificing anything.

We had a lot of barbecues over the holidays, too, and they were great fun. I kept well away from sausages because they are very fatty, but I'd have a small piece of grilled steak and I'd pile my plate with different salads.

I started to find that the less I ate fatty food, the less I craved it. If I ate something fatty I would taste it immediately and it was a real turnoff.

When we got home from holidays, the first thing I did was jump on the scales. I was 212 pounds; I hadn't budged and that was wonderful news. I'd managed to survive Christmas and New Year's without putting on any weight.

The less I ate fatty food, the less I craved it.

I set more goals for myself for the New Year. I walked more, and I did more sit-ups. I pushed myself a bit further and a bit further again. If I felt comfortable, I'd double my walk. It was summer and such beautiful weather, so I'd walk as far as I could. But I only did it while I enjoyed it. I never pushed myself too hard; if I didn't enjoy walking for longer I didn't do it.

A World of Difference

I really started to feel at ease while I was walking. Feeling the sun on my skin was relaxing. I began to see the world through different eyes. That time alone with my thoughts made me appreciate the world around me. I saw things I'd never seen as an obese person. It was a time of real spiritual growth for me—it gave me time to contemplate my life.

I loved having the wind blowing my hair and the sun on my skin. I'd never really felt these things before. During the solitude of my walks I felt I was getting in touch with myself.

I had really started to believe in myself and my own ability. I actually believed I had the courage to achieve my goals. That was a very different mind-set for me because in the past I'd always had doubts in the back of my mind.

For the first time in my life I was really at peace with myself. The mental struggles that had burdened me for years were gone. I felt like I had the power to direct my life—I had never felt that before. I could really feel the power of believing in myself. I had control. That was a huge step for me.

I felt I had so much to live for now and I looked forward to getting up in the morning.

Feeling this way actually gave me more energy, too. I wasn't wallowing in feeling sorry for myself anymore. I knew in my heart that my life was worth living.

I stopped yelling at the kids over small things, which just didn't seem important. Instead of yelling at them, I wanted to do more with them and spend more time with my husband. I wanted to see my kids laugh and play, and I wanted to laugh and play with them. We talked a lot more at home, too.

I used to take things very much to heart, but I won't let people put me down anymore. Now I ignore negative comments and think, *Well, everybody's different.* I no longer get overwhelmed by a sideways stare or a snicker. Before, the simplest hurtful comment could destroy me for a week; now I look at the people who make such comments and think, *Isn't it sad they are so negative about life.*

Jason didn't watch what he was eating at all. He ate what he wanted to, but because I'd changed what we ate and how I cooked, he lost weight, too.

He'd lost thirty pounds without even trying. He ate as much as he'd always eaten but now his meals were healthy.

I felt I had so much to live for now; I was really doing something worthwhile with my life and I looked forward to getting up in the morning.

We loved going to the park with the kids and kicking the soccer ball around. Often the kids would say "Stop, Mum, we need to rest," and they'd sit down for a few minutes while I was still ready to play. What a change!

The first day I wore size 16 pants, I was so happy I cried.

Jason and I became more intimate and more passionate. My emotions had changed, which helped us feel much closer. It was probably because I was becoming proud of my body instead of ashamed.

It got to the stage where my weight-loss program wasn't even a conscious effort, it had just become a part of my day-to-day routine. I no longer had to think about what I ate, I just ate the foods I had been cooking.

My goal weight was 165 pounds. That's what my doctor and I had worked out to be a healthy, safe weight. When I got to around 175 pounds I knew I was well on my way. We'd been invited to a friend's wedding and it was my target to get down to 170 pounds. I had six weeks to lose the weight, and after that I was only a few pounds away from my goal weight.

I felt like I could conquer the world.

I had thrown out all of my "fat" clothes by then. I was wearing a size 16! The first day I wore size 16 pants, I was so happy I cried.

I was going to wear the dress I'd worn for New Year's Eve to my friend's wedding, so I took it to the shop a few weeks beforehand to have it taken in. It felt good, and on the day of the wedding I weighed myself—I had reached 170 pounds.

Each time I achieved a goal I felt immensely rewarded. Each target I achieved gave me the courage to continue, and the inspiration to reach the next target.

I felt like I could conquer the world.

"I can finally enjoy being a grandmother."

Lina

Starting Weight: **203** pounds

Current Weight: **143** pounds

60 POUNDS LOST!

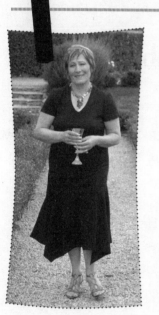

I had a small but very important reason to lose weight: my two-year-old granddaughter. At 203 pounds, I struggled to play with her. I had no energy to keep up with her and I wasn't able to enjoy my time with her; it was terrible and made me so unhappy. I couldn't fit into my clothes and I knew in my heart it was time to change. I'd been putting on weight slowly for years, so busy raising my family and looking after everyone else that I stopped looking after myself. Now it was time for me.

I have lost 60 pounds and totally regained my enthusiasm for life. I feel younger, and physically I feel fantastic. I have more energy than I've had in years. It took me two years to lose the weight, but I'm so proud of myself for sticking to it. And when I look back at how different my life is, I know it was well worth the effort. I'm very happy to leave the old me behind.

CHAPTER SIX

Farewell, Flab!

TWO WEEKS LATER I JUMPED ON THE SCALES AND, BINGO, I HAD reached my goal weight—165 pounds. It was June 5, 2000—I will remember that day as one of the happiest of my life.

I cried out to Jason from the bathroom and when he saw me on the scales he knew straight away why I was yelling. He scooped me up in his arms and spun me around in the air. The emotion that we felt then was intense. I had done it—after thirteen months I had reached my goal! I was so proud. My boys came running in—they couldn't understand why I was crying. I had to explain to them that Mummy was crying because she was happy, not sad!

> *I had done it—after thirteen months I had reached my goal.*

I ran across to my parents' house and told them; Mum cried and Dad hugged me. They were full of admiration for what I'd achieved.

Jason took me out for dinner that night and we celebrated. I was on cloud nine; it was the most amazing feeling of my life. I had done this all on my own. I had begun to have faith in myself and won the biggest battle of my life.

I'm not an educated person, I'm not a doctor or a dietician. I'm just a mum who made her dream come true.

I wore a pair of pants out to dinner and I looked and felt like a million dollars. I felt like a real woman for the first time in my life, and I really thought I was the luckiest person in the world. But more than anything I was truly happy with myself—I was not an obese person any longer. We were at a restaurant eating dinner and no one was staring at me. I walked in with my head up high and my shoulders back, and I felt good.

The Last Step to My New Life

Getting to my goal weight was a dream come true, but because I'd been so overweight for so long, I had a lot of excess skin left after the weight loss. I couldn't wear jeans because, while I was happy with what I'd achieved, I was still a little paranoid about the loose flap of skin around my waist.

I spoke with my doctor to see what could be done. He explained that my skin had been so stretched for so long, the elasticity was gone and there was little hope of getting rid of it on my own. The only option would be to have surgery to remove the excess skin. I was very conflicted—the thought of needing surgery was disheartening after all the hard work I'd put into losing weight. At the same time, I'd come so far on this journey and worked so hard to lose weight that I didn't want to still be self-conscious of my body.

I'm not an educated person, I'm not a doctor or a dietician. I'm just a mum who made her dream come true.

After much consideration, I finally agreed to have the operation. I was terrified the day of the operation, but I had Jason and my family to keep me strong. The surgery was very painful—ten times worse than childbirth—and it took me three months to recover. But when the stitches healed and I was able to see my new body for the first time, I knew then that the battle was completely over. Everything that I'd wanted to achieve, I had. The final step was done. The excess skin weighed 10 pounds and, for the first time in my life, I could look at myself naked and feel not just comfortable, but incredibly confident and proud!

My First Pair of Jeans

Because I'd always been overweight, I'd never, ever worn a pair of jeans. I'd dreamed of the day I'd be able to go into a store and buy my first pair of jeans off the rack. I was at my cousin's house one afternoon and she told me she'd just bought jeans—size 12. She asked me if I wanted to try them on. I was so reluctant, especially a size 12! But she said, "Go for it."

I went into her bedroom on my own and put them on. They were great. Every button did up and they fit perfectly—I was wearing size 12 jeans. I sat on the end of her bed and cried with happiness. I stayed in there for about fifteen minutes before I decided to go out and show them. When I walked out, Jason shed tears, too. He knew how much this meant to me. They were all excited for me because they knew what I'd been through to get there.

I was wearing size 12 jeans. I sat on the end of her bed and cried with happiness.

We arranged for her to come with me the next day to buy myself a pair of jeans. And I did. Every time I put those jeans on I remember how hard I had to work to get into them. It still means so much to me to be able to wear them.

After I bought my jeans, we went out to celebrate. I bought a new pair of high heels, and I wore a tight black top with a dinner jacket—I knew I looked amazing and Jason told me I looked gorgeous.

I was on cloud nine.

I went through a stage when I just lived in my bathtub—I hadn't been able to have a bath before I'd lost my weight because I couldn't fit! So it was a real luxury for me to run a bath full of beautiful oils and bubble bath and just lie there thinking about my life and reflecting on what I'd achieved. It felt incredibly good. I would stay there thinking about people's reactions to me now in comparison with how they had acted before.

Every time I put those jeans on I remember how hard I had to work to get into them.

On those nights I just lay there in the bath, staring at my body, sometimes for more than an hour, and for a while I found it difficult to get used to what I saw. I loved my new shape but for so long I had never been able to imagine that I'd be a slim woman, yet here I was. Was this really my body before me?

I'd picture all the food I used to eat—the chocolate bars, the pizza, the mashed potatoes drowned in butter, the chips and burgers—and then I'd compare them with what I ate today.

I just can't believe how different my life is. The most amazing thing was watching people's reactions. It was as if I'd been away on a desert island for twelve months—the looks on their faces! They were seeing the real Karen for the first time ever.

Some people didn't even recognize me. The man who lived across the road from us thought Jason was having an affair. He was—but with his own wife!

Through all of this, I was determined that my personality wouldn't change. I wanted a new body but I wanted the same me inside. And I haven't changed, although I do see life through different eyes and am much calmer. I believe I'm much more tolerant, too. But the nicest thing is that my husband and my family love me for who I am, not how I look.

Shopping for clothes is now something I can enjoy. I can walk into any shop I like and buy anything. That was a whole new experience for me. Simple things that other women take for granted have become an important part of my life and my confidence has grown day by day.

After I lost the weight, I became so excited about going out. I loved seeing myself in beautiful clothes and I loved getting ready to go out. Before, I'd dreaded getting ready, I'd hated it. I could spend two hours doing my hair and makeup and still feel desperately ugly. Now, it was a pleasure.

Even though I was at my goal weight I still kept walking every day. But, having gotten to the stage where I had reached my goal weight, I didn't want losing weight to become an obsession for me. I didn't want dieting to control my life. I allowed myself four or five pounds "to play with." If I put on a few extra pounds it was okay. I ate the same healthy food, but if I felt like a piece of chocolate or we took the kids out for pizza, it was okay for me to join in.

I'm in a world of maintaining now, that's the level I'm at. There's no way I'm going to go back to my bad habits, but I'm enjoying food. I eat in moderation, and I eat well. I weigh myself about once a week now and I don't get stressed.

I am grateful for every single day and every single opportunity that comes my way.

Sharing the Clothesline Diet

Jason and I were sitting together one night when he said, "Karen, I think there's still one more goal we have to achieve together—to rebuild our dream house." He was right. Our earlier traumas had virtually robbed us of our first home and I really never thought we'd ever be able to build something like that again.

Jason and I wanted to stay in the same area, and there was a new development that had opened up about a five-minute drive away. We wanted to be close to my mum and dad and this lot was a twenty-minute walk away from them; I could walk there easily.

We put a deposit down on the lot and got in touch with a few local real-estate agents to sell our house. Three gave us their valuations. We were thrilled with their quotes and decided to put the house on the market that day.

Six days later the house was sold! I couldn't believe it, I was still trying to adjust to us selling it, and it was already gone.

We were a little sad on the day we had to leave the house we'd sold. I cried on the doorstep when we left for the final time. That house had given us so much joy, but we were looking forward to our new life in a new house.

I felt guilty for leaving my clothesline behind, since it had been so much a part of my weight loss. After we moved I went back to our old house and approached the new owners—I was on a mission to get my clothesline back! I asked them if I could buy it from them and explained what it meant to me. Without hesitation, they agreed to my request. I now have it stored away safely. That clothesline and I had gone through far too much together to be apart now!

One evening Jason and the boys were sitting on the couch watching television. I was in the kitchen washing the dishes when Jason called out to come to the living room quickly.

There was a story on television about a woman who'd lost 130 pounds. Naturally I was like a sponge when it came to weight-loss stories; I read and watched every one I could.

The woman had undergone a stomach stapling operation that had ended badly. Her stomach had been stapled too small and she spent four months in hospital eating food through a drip while she recovered, yet she still talked glowingly about how wonderful her new life was as a skinny person.

I was furious! It really bothered me to think that the message was being sent out that this was a good way to lose weight. Jason suggested I ring the TV station and tell them how irresponsible the story was—so I did! I told them how I'd lost my weight and they were so excited they came out to film me! I was determined to show obese people that you can do it on your own. The story went to air and began a roller-coaster ride for me. I asked them to include my number so that anyone wanting help could call me. I thought I'd be lucky if ten people phoned. Well, the phone rang and rang. By the time I'd hang up my voice mail was full again. The local papers rang, a major national magazine rang and I had people calling me at home wanting my help. I was thrilled at the response; I had more than four hundred phone calls. With every call I first explained to them that I wasn't a professional or a dietician or doctor. I was just a mum who'd lost a lot of weight. My mailbox was full every day—it was fantastic! I replied to every single letter personally. My mum suggested we convert her laundry into an office. Some days there were bags and bags of mail on the floor while poor Mum was doing the washing around me.

Two years earlier I'd been wishing I were dead, now I was on top of the world.

I had so many calls from so many people wanting help I decided to hold a public meeting to address everyone. I was going to have them all at home for coffee, but I got six hundred and fifty requests and I couldn't fit everyone in my backyard! Two years earlier I'd been wishing I were dead, now I was on top of the world.

The magazine wanted to do a photo shoot with me, and they'd arrange for me to go to a beautiful hotel in the city to have my hair and makeup done and be photographed. I'd heard of this hotel but never dared to go inside it! I was so excited—I felt like a princess. It was so beautiful—marble floors, polished silver staircase—Jason and I were mesmerized, it was so far out of our world. That day was magical and I couldn't wait for the magazine to hit the stands, but it was quickly back to reality; I had a public talk to organize.

All the details were arranged, the hall booked. I'd organized tea and coffee for everyone and I couldn't wait to meet all of the people I'd spoken to over the phone. I knew in my heart I could help them, but my greatest fear was that when they realized I wasn't educated they wouldn't listen to me. I wasn't a weight-loss expert. I'd only lost weight myself. I was nervous no one would turn up, but the room was full. While I spoke they all sat silently. Then came dozens of questions. I answered everyone without having to think twice; the answers just rolled off my tongue. When we finished, they applauded. It was the first time in my life I had truly been heard and the first time in my life I felt important. The response was so overwhelming we did it again the next week, and the week after. And we've been doing it weekly ever since!

As I lay in bed that night, I felt totally free and in control of my life and my future, and I knew what I wanted to do with my life. I wanted desperately to help free all of those people who have struggled with their weight the way I have.

My support group meets every week and I have done talks all over Australia and the United States. Our group has lost thousands of pounds and I am so proud of everyone who has taken the steps to change their life. I still get excited when I hear their inspiring success stories.

That incredible response prompted me to write *The Clothesline Diet*. So many people were searching for the same answers I had been searching for, but I'd found them and I knew my story could help others. So we wrote *The Clothesline Diet*.

When *The Clothesline Diet* was finally published my life took another new turn. We counted down each day until the book hit the stands and it gave me such a great thrill to finally see it on display. On the morning the book was released I raced into the local shopping center and there it was. Seeing it, I had butterflies in my stomach. I spent the whole day going from shop to shop seeing if the book was on the shelves. Everywhere I went I saw it. I couldn't believe it! I'm so proud and it's still a thrill today when I see the book or when people approach me and say hello or that they've read the book. I love hearing their stories and hearing what they thought about my story.

> *I wanted desperately to help free all of those people who have struggled with their weight the way I have.*

About three weeks after the book went on sale I took the usual trip to the mailbox, but there was just a little card inside telling me I had to collect my mail from the counter.

When I went inside the postal officer laughed at me and said, "Are you ready for this?" Then he lifted several huge bags onto the counter. I couldn't believe they were for me! Each bag was full of letters. I started crying in the middle of the post office! I rang Jason straightaway and cried on the phone to him, I was so excited. From that point on the mail has never stopped coming, and every day I love going to the mailbox to read about other people's experiences with weight loss. I love hearing their stories, and with every letter I feel as if I've come to know the person who's written me. It's a real privilege to be a part of people's lives, to share their ups and downs.

My dream is the same as it was after I lost my weight; that is, to help others do the same. For someone like me to have achieved what I have really proved to me that anyone can achieve anything, and that's the message I want to share. You can accomplish anything if you believe in yourself. I respond to every single letter and though it can take me a little while to get back to everybody, I do my best.

My Happily Ever After

The day finally arrived for us to move into our new house. What an incredible feeling! We moved in on a Friday and by Sunday night Jason and I had unpacked everything and settled in. The last room to be arranged was my new study. Jason got a desk from work that he polished up—it's just beautiful—and we put up pictures of the people in my support group. I love that room—it's my little space in the house where I can be me and escape. It's in that room that I sit and read about people's problems in the letters they've sent me. Some days I can't even fit all the mail on the desk.

Dreams don't come knocking on your door. You have to turn your dreams into reality.

Being in the house is a dream come true—I'm in my own beautiful home, married to the man I love and adore and have two precious boys. What more could I ask for? I feel as if I am the luckiest person alive. But when I think about it realistically, everything I have today, from my house to Jason and the boys, was something I had to fight for. And my weight, of course, was the biggest battle—the biggest journey of my life.

Dreams don't come knocking on your door. You have to turn your dreams into reality. I wanted children so badly, I was so desperate, and I fought and fought and it happened. It's taken us seven years to rebuild our dream home, but we did that, too. Losing my weight was a thirteen-month battle, and every day presented a new challenge, but I did it. I kept fighting and I did it. Now everything I have today, my friends, my family, I thank God for.

I thank God for giving me the belief in myself. It's up to us to make life work, to make a dream become reality, a fantasy become real.

The best piece of advice I can give is this: if you're not happy with your life, change it. It's never, ever too late to change your life. I'm not a doctor or a dietician, I'm just an everyday, average mum. I changed my life myself—nobody else did it for me.

> *The best piece of advice I can give is this: if you're not happy with your life, change it. It's never, ever too late to change your life.*

For years friends and family have been encouraging Jason and me to renew our vows. I'd never really given it a thought; we were married and that was it. But after hearing it over and over, Jason and I began talking about it and decided it was a great idea.

We were at Mum and Dad's one night soon after we'd decided to remarry and I slipped into Mum's room and pulled out my old wedding dress—it was huge! As I was feeling the beads and the lace I broke out in goose bumps. I had to put it on. Oh, my god! How different I looked. I was standing in my dress looking in the same mirror I'd looked in thirteen years ago on my wedding day. I burst into tears. I couldn't believe the transformation my whole life had undergone.

> *I burst into tears. I couldn't believe the transformation my whole life had undergone.*

We set the date for March 16 and I was excited to start planning. I truly couldn't remember being as excited the first time around! I couldn't imagine wearing any wedding dress but my first, but at a size 32, it had a long way to go before it would fit me now. I took the dress to a designer and tried it on for her. I walked out of the dressing room and stood in front of the mirror with this huge dress hanging off me. The designer grabbed the big, puffy sleeves and with a flick of her scissors, they were gone! Within seconds, my new dress started to come to life.

A week later, we went back to the designer. When she carried the dress out of the fitting room, Mum burst into tears. I put it on and I couldn't believe how beautiful it was. I couldn't wait to see Jason's face when I made my way down the aisle.

On the Saturday night before our second wedding, as I was packing a few things from the bathroom to take to Mum and Dad's, I jumped on the scales for the first time in a while. The numbers flickered to 155 pounds. I didn't want to compare this second wedding with our first but I couldn't help it—I was almost *half* the size I was on my original wedding day. Half the size and twice as happy!

I was almost half the size I was on my original wedding day. Half the size and twice as happy!

On the day of the ceremony, I felt the way I had thirteen years ago, as if I was leaving Mum and Dad for the very first time. All through the day, I was reliving my first wedding, with one magical difference—this time I was overwhelmed with excitement and delight, not anguish. I hated getting ready for my first wedding because I hated myself and how I looked so much. This time, I felt proud, confident and beautiful. I felt like a true bride—the way I should have felt the first time around.

As I walked down the aisle toward Jason, I could see how nervous and excited he was, too. He later told me that his heart was pounding like mad and when he caught sight of me, everything else around him disappeared—he thought I looked that beautiful!

When I took Jason's hand during the ceremony, I was overwhelmed with happiness that we had the opportunity to celebrate our love all over again. It was as if God has given us a chance to start our lives over. We knew what we'd been through to get to this day: losing our home, losing each other, struggling for children, struggling with my weight. We'd had many heartaches, but every heartache was worth it to get to where we are today. The best part of all was that we had everyone who had supported us along the way in one room. Our friends, our family, the support group, all of the people we loved.

If you believe in yourself you can make any dream come true—and you can. All you need is the courage to take that very first step.

After the ceremony, we made our way down a set of stairs toward Brendan and Ryan, who were holding a ribbon for us to cut and walk through.

Thirteen years ago, I'd agonized over walking through that bridal arch, terrified that we'd get stuck underneath it together because I was so big. For our renewal, we had two massive candelabras set up as an entranceway, strung together with a ribbon that we were to cut and walk through. This time, Jason and I walked proudly, side by side. For me, this ribbon was symbolic of a new beginning. When we cut it and walked through without hesitation, I truly understood how far I'd come—how far we'd come—since first starting my journey.

I always say that if you believe in yourself you can make any dream come true—and you can. All you need is the courage to take that very first step.

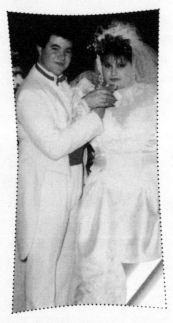

Our first wedding

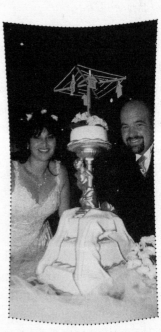

Renewing our vows with a touch of the Clothesline

> ## "If I hadn't been sacked I might very well be dead right now."
>
> ### Richard
>
> Starting Weight: **390** pounds
>
> Current Weight: **290** pounds
>
> # 100 POUNDS LOST!

I knew I had to lose weight. The need to lose weight really bites you on the bum when you can barely lift your bum off the ground! The scales told me I was 390 pounds, so heavy that I was struggling to walk.

But life's funny, isn't it? I knew in my heart that I really needed to lose weight, but I still don't think I would have done it had I not been sacked.

I was fired from my job as a postal worker because I was too fat. In hindsight it probably saved my life.

My weight began to pile on immediately after my wife left. I was eating a lot of bad food and drinking very heavily. I was lonely and bored and hated being alone, so I went to the pub for company. My heart was heavy all the time and I felt a complete and overwhelming sense of hopelessness, total hopelessness.

My weight grew at a monstrous rate. I'd really lost control over my whole life and I began to suffer depression very badly. I was quite a happy, jovial bloke beforehand, but life did an about-face on me.

My weight and my depression grew until I was under a cloud of darkness I couldn't budge. It didn't sink in that I really could lose my weight until I met Karen. Karen showed me how much weight she'd lost and how she'd done it. I couldn't believe that I was looking at the same person I'd seen in pictures!

We had a good long talk about my weight, and she gave me the confidence to believe I could do it. After all, if she'd done it, why couldn't I?

My diet changed quite a bit after I met Karen. I was a single man—I never cooked and I had no idea about what food was right and what was wrong. I didn't have recipe books at home or a wife to cook me healthy meals.

Karen took me shopping at my local market. As we walked through the fruit and veggie aisles, we talked about what was good and what was bad. It was a big learning experience for me. I really soaked up the information she gave me because I believed her. I felt like I could trust her.

I began by walking in the water at the pool. It was hard work; every morning I'd leave my house at 7:00 a.m., drive to the pool and walk up and down from one side of the pool to the other, for as long as I could. I started doing it for ten minutes, then fifteen minutes, then I got up to half an hour.

The first time I stepped into that pool, I thought I was going to die. Aside from the sheer embarrassment of being in a suit at my size, it was bloody hard work just getting in and out of the pool! But the weight began to move and with each little step my confidence grew. My life has changed so much I barely know how to describe it.

I can walk for miles now and I can dance. I'm so much more outgoing.

I've amazed myself with how well I'm doing, and I'm so proud. I've still got a long way to go to reach my goal weight of 200 pounds, but I've come a long way and the hardest part of the journey is behind me. Karen has changed my life, physically and mentally. Her spirit's so infectious you just can't help but catch her enthusiasm and optimism. She had faith in me and that gave me faith in myself.

The Clothesline Diet Bible

Change Your Life, One Step at a Time

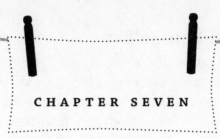

CHAPTER SEVEN

Getting Started:

Taking the First Steps to Your New Life

· ·

PART TWO OF THIS BOOK IS WHAT I CALL THE DIET BIBLE. THIS
section includes everything you really need to know about losing your weight
for good—and it's based on tried and tested solutions, solutions that worked
for me and have worked for thousands of others. And believe me, after twenty
years of dieting, I've tried everything with no results, but this really works.

In the following pages you'll find practical ways to keep your motivation and
rebuild your self-esteem (no more "start on Monday finish on Tuesday" diets!):

- my super-easy seven-day diet plan

- my step-by-step exercise guide

- some of my favorite, healthy (and easy-to-make) recipes

- honest answers to questions every dieter asks, with helpful tips I
  learned along the way

It's all at your fingertips, it's all easy to understand and it's all information
that I collected while I was searching for answers to my problems. Keep this
book with you, copy pages if you need to. Stick them to the fridge, in your diary,
behind the bathroom door! Keep it on hand and whenever you need a little
guidance, I'm with you. I've done it, you can, too, so no more excuses. Make like
a kangaroo and hop to it! You've got nothing to lose but a whole lot of fat!

Believing in Yourself

Every dieter knows that one of the biggest battles is keeping motivated, especially if you have low self-esteem to start with. Who hasn't started a diet on Monday and given up by Friday (or in my case Monday afternoon!)—a diet where all you've lost is tons of confidence. It's really hard to fight temptation—it's easier to give in and say, "One cookie won't hurt," or "I don't deserve this. I can't do it. I'll never lose weight." And before you know it, half a packet of cookies are gone (straight to your thighs) and your diet is over before it began. So, here's how I did it: it's all about having a shoulder to cry on, taking control of your life and putting yourself first. But first of all, it's about believing in yourself, because you can do it. You *can*. And you deserve this.

It's about believing in yourself, because you can do it. You can. And you deserve this.

Low self-esteem is one of the most important factors to overcome in order to achieve weight loss. It's a topic we address frequently in my support groups. Everybody in the group writes their answers to the questions: What is the meaning of low self-esteem? And what is the cause of it?

Before you can move on with your life, you need to improve your self-esteem—you have the power within you to do so.

If you can answer these questions, then you clearly know the reason for your low self-esteem. So the question then remains—you know how the problem has arisen, so why aren't you addressing it? Before you can move on with your life, you need to improve your self-esteem—you have the power within you to do so.

I didn't need anyone else to hate me— I had enough hate for everyone.

When I was at my heaviest, I had terribly low self-esteem. My self-confidence was at rock bottom. People were constantly putting me down, and I felt worthless. But the truth is that low self-esteem comes from within, and makes you criticize yourself constantly. I had a repeating loop of thoughts that were always with me: a little voice in my head saying, "You don't belong in this world," "You're good for nothing," "Nobody likes you like this," "You're a terrible mother and wife," "You're ugly and disgusting." And these were my feelings toward myself!

I didn't need anyone else to hate me—I had enough hate for everyone. I would always compare myself negatively to others and feel intimidated because I wasn't as educated or I didn't have a particular talent. I felt that I was never good enough and I believed I was a failure at everything I tried to accomplish—before I'd even tried to accomplish it!

When I was at rock bottom and decided to change my life, I knew I had to change each and every negative thought I had about myself. I fought the negative voice in my head and I won. I took each negative thought, turned it around and reminded myself that I deserved a better life. The key was proving to myself that my mind was the one wreaking havoc on my heart and my feelings; nobody else. Now that I am more confident, no amount of criticizing will wither my self-esteem. No one can turn all of the positives that I have worked so hard for back into negatives. I have full control over my thoughts.

No one can turn all of the positives that I have worked so hard for back into negatives.

Having low self-esteem and feeling unhappy with yourself is common. But it *can* be beaten. If you believe in yourself, you can overcome that negativity. And once you do, you'll lose weight more easily and see your goals more clearly. I used to give myself a small exercise every night before I went to bed. I'd stand in front of the mirror and look myself in the eye and say, "I deserve a better life, I want a better life, I can do this. Karen, you can do this." I'd repeat it each and every night, and eventually I broke through all the negative thoughts and let all the positive ones in.

I had to learn to treat myself the way I had always treated others.

Another exercise you can try is called "give yourself credit." If you don't reward yourself for your accomplishments, you begin to degrade yourself. I always degraded myself because I looked for approval from others. I was ashamed and insecure about the choices I made in life, so I constantly sought the approval of others. But now I concentrate on giving myself a pat on the back and following my heart. I trust in myself to make decisions and if I make a bad decision, what does it matter? Nobody is perfect, we all have failings and that's perfectly okay.

Learning a little patience was one of the hardest things to do. I had to accept that it would take time to achieve my goals. Realizing your dreams doesn't come easily, and I recognized that I had to be proud of what I'd achieved at every step along the way and acknowledge how far I'd come in order to stay motivated.

It's an old adage, but one of the greatest rules in life is to treat others the way you expect to be treated yourself—I had to learn to treat *myself* the way I had always treated others. Giving myself a little bit of credit isn't that hard at all now.

Getting the Support You Need

Everybody needs a shoulder to cry on, someone who will listen and be there during the tough times. I will be that shoulder to cry on for you, but I also want you to look around you and pick someone close to you who will be your support buddy when you need it. Maybe it's your husband, your wife, a neighbor, a friend. You're not asking them to go on the diet with you; you're just asking them for their unconditional support. Confide in them how you truly feel about yourself and why you want to lose weight, and I know you will find that support you need.

When I started my diet, Jason had no idea just how low my life was until I sat him down, talked to him and asked him to be a part of my journey. He'd never really understood the depth of my despair because I'd never told him. I'd always put on a brave face and we'd joke about how I'd start a new diet every week, but deep down I wasn't laughing. So this time, I explained to him why this was important to me and why I needed to change my life. It was the first time I acknowledged *Setting up your own support network is crucial.* to him that I knew I had a weight problem, and from that moment he was my rock, no questions asked. Instead of complaining that there was no soda in the fridge and only low-fat cookies in the cupboard, he encouraged me and he shared every small triumph along the way. Setting up your own support network is crucial.

Many times I felt so alone in my battle to beat my weight that I would have loved having someone to talk to, someone who truly understood what I was going through and who could guide me when times were dark. That's why I started my support group. We meet every Monday night at a local community center: we talk, we cry and we have formed friendships that will last forever. We begin by walking for twenty minutes or so in small circles around the room (this way those who are struggling can take a break without feeling bad). We power walk in each session usually around the room at the center but sometimes on late summer days we

walk on the nearby track. I can see them all talking and chatting to one another and before they know it, everyone has walked for half an hour without realizing they're actually exercising!

> *The secret to losing weight is taking control of your life.*

Then we swap recipes, talk and share our stories, laugh and cry. Some weeks we have an instructor who teaches basic Tae Bo and kickboxing, and other weeks we learn self-defense or line dancing. We want to promote activity to show everyone that there's so much of life to enjoy, and most of all we want to show that exercise can be an enjoyable part of life, not a chore.

Anyone can set up their own support group. Look around you, talk to people in your neighborhood, talk to your friends. We all know someone who wants to lose weight, right? How does the old saying go? "A problem shared is a problem halved."

Taking Control of Your Life

No matter where I speak, the message is always the same: the secret to losing weight is taking control of your life. Losing weight successfully isn't just about dieting. You need to stand up for yourself, take control of your life and stop letting life—whether it's work pressure, family pressure or food—control you.

Make time for yourself. Give yourself the time to go for a little walk around the block to clear your head. Life is a challenge for everybody; we all have our hurdles to overcome, whether it's balancing work and family, making time for your relationships, finding time for the kids, paying off the mortgage or credit cards, or all of the above.

It's vital that we take each problem that life throws at us step-by-step, take each day as it comes and work through it. Nowadays, we hear and read a lot about depression. Depression is one of the biggest issues that arises in our support groups and in the letters I receive. Despite the fact that materially we're better off than we've ever been before, there seems to be an epidemic of people suffering from depression. For our parents and grandparents, life was a whole lot tougher than it is for our generation. We have everything at our fingertips—refrigerators, toasters, DVDs, cars, clothes—all the material things we could ever dream of. So why are we so depressed?

I suffered from terrible depression for years (perhaps even decades!). My weight was a major factor contributing to the depression, of course. My self-esteem had all but gone and I hated myself. I honestly had days where I felt so bad I convinced myself I had nothing to live for. But I believe I was so depressed because I was so busy concentrating on small things around me, like making sure my house was clean by a certain time every day, making sure my washing was done by a certain time and that my kids were fed by a certain time, and making sure I was there for my husband when he got home each day. I spent all day worrying about all of these tasks and all of the other people in my life. But what about me? The bottom line was, there was never any time left for me to take care of myself.

When I began to put aside a few minutes for myself, I began to feel that I was gaining control of my life again.

When I began to put aside a few minutes for myself, even for the simplest things—a bubble bath, painting my nails or a cup of coffee while I read a magazine—I began to feel that I was gaining control of my life again. If the washing wasn't done by 3:00 p.m. on Tuesday, it wasn't the end of the world. It could be done the next day, what did it matter? I live a different life now, in the sense that I have the confidence within me to do the things I want to do, rather than what I think I have to do.

We complain far too easily about our lives and yet, if we just take a minute and think, we see how privileged we really are.

People have ups and downs in their lives, often more downs than ups, and that's life. But when those downs happen, we can change the way we think about them to keep depression from setting in.

At my support group we talk a lot about why and how life becomes too much for people. As a group, we discuss our problems and, together, work to turn those negatives into positives. Something that comes up often is the way we can take life for granted. We don't appreciate the time, the day or one another. We complain because we have a cold or a headache, but what about people who are truly physically suffering? We complain that we have no money, we're always broke, but what about the people who have no food, who have nowhere to live? We complain that we can't be bothered going for a walk or cleaning the house; what about those people who are physically impaired and would relish the chance to simply take a walk in the sunshine?

We complain far too easily about our lives and yet, if we just take a minute and think, we see how privileged we really are. We don't appreciate the simple things that we have: food, shelter, clothing, family. We have clean water when we turn on a tap. We flick a switch and have electricity. We open the fridge and there's food there.

Turning your negative thoughts into positive ones is the single most essential factor in changing your life.

The bottom line is that life's too short to worry about trivial problems every day. You must find peace within yourself and start enjoying every minute you have. When you have full control over yourself, you will have full control over your life. A lot of people turn to food when they are feeling down, depressed or stressed, and eating for comfort, or emotional eating, is the biggest factor in weight gain. It certainly was for me.

I truly believe that turning your negative thoughts into positive ones is the single most essential factor in changing your life. When I started to take control and change my attitude toward day-to-day problems, the problems seemed less significant and much of the stress disappeared. Instead of allowing problems to accumulate and grow in my mind, I turned each problem from a negative to a positive. Instead of thinking the world was caving in on me—that life was controlling me—I took charge and faced the problem head-on, and then got on with my life. And I felt good about that. Instead of feeling depressed, I felt great that I had handled the problem rather than letting it handle me.

For example, now if I have an argument with Jason, instead of bottling up my feelings and stewing on the fight for days, which I used to do, I confront it and move on. If that means I have to back down or we both have to compromise a little, it doesn't matter—as long as we resolve it. We're stronger for it as a couple, and I'm stronger for it as a person.

Once you turn the negative factors in your life into positives, you'll find the weight comes off much more quickly and much more easily. Realistically, my weight loss wasn't just because of my diet, it was because I decided to change my life. The diet was just the means to make the change happen.

Putting Yourself First

To make any significant change work, you have to look deep within yourself. I didn't wake up that morning after the Mother's Day dance saying, "Okay, I'm going to lose 150 pounds in a year." I had to start from scratch and work through a lot of issues. I had to overcome all of the negative voices in my head saying, "It's too late in life to lose weight," "You don't deserve this," "You'll never stick to it," before I could even begin. I had to take full control and accept that I was number one, not number three or four, in my life.

> *My weight loss wasn't just because of my diet, it was because I decided to change my life. The diet was just the means to make the change happen.*

It's essential that you put yourself first in life. I know that I have a husband and two children who I care for deeply, but I still need to be first on my list. If I don't make me number one, my kids are not going to have a good mother and my husband is not going to have a good wife.

Years ago, I was number three. My kids were my first priority, then my husband, then me, and I was always depressed. I was always yelling at the kids, screaming at them to have a bath or go to bed. I was like a constantly erupting volcano. But when I taught myself to be number one in my life, I found I was—and still am—much calmer within myself and in my approach to life. Now, if the boys don't pack their toys away, instead of yelling the roof off, I speak to them calmly about it and they respond. Making myself the number one priority changed my whole family's life for the better.

> *It's essential that you put yourself first in life.*

Back then, when I was totally depressed and weighed in at 300 pounds, I had no life. And because I didn't have a life, I made my kids' and my husband's lives absolute hell. They were depressed because I was depressed. But when I began to make myself a priority, these problems seemed to melt away.

When you can see your life clearly, you can achieve any goal you set your mind to. As long as you have a dream, an image in your mind, you can achieve it because your heart will fight for dreams. I have watched people's relationships with their children, their husbands, wives, other family and friends change and go from strength to strength when they begin to put themselves first. They can see their relationships through totally different eyes.

There truly is only one person who can change your life—you.

With every step toward your goal weight, you will find you achieved so much more along the way than just weight loss.

There is no doctor or dietician, no pill and no potion that can heal you from within. You must achieve this yourself, and you can. There truly is only one person who can change your life—you. When you begin to believe in yourself, you will begin to see a lot of positive things happen. Your life will feel more purpose driven, and you'll begin to appreciate every single day. You will also find that your weight will come off much more quickly. You will love waking up each morning and, with every step toward your goal weight, you will find you achieved so much more along the way than just weight loss.

Don't Give Up!

I spent so many years waiting to lose weight because, in all honesty, I never truly gave myself the chance to try. Why do we sometimes fail before we've even begun? The answer is simple—because we are afraid that we will fail. We'd rather not begin at all than begin and fail. We don't have the necessary faith in ourselves to go out on that limb and try to achieve our goals. We allow doubts to creep into our minds and fester.

Don't give up before you've even begun— throw yourself at life and enjoy the journey.

The truth is that life is so short there isn't a moment to waste. I don't want to die with any doubts or lingering guilt about all I had left to achieve. Even if I try at something and it doesn't work out, I won't be disappointed as long as I know I've given life my best shot. Don't give up before you've even begun—throw yourself at life and enjoy the journey.

When we speak about this in our support group, everyone nods in empathy. And thanks to the work we're doing, I've really seen such changes in the personalities of everyone who has walked through the doors of my support group. I've seen them blossom and embrace life and I can't tell you how proud that makes me. I see them go from being shy, overweight people who really don't enjoy life at all, to being vibrant, energetic lovers of it. They are becoming the people they have always dreamed of being. The transformation is unbelievable and so rewarding. It's almost like watching butterflies emerge from their cocoons!

No matter how hard I tried I wasn't satisfied with my life because I wasn't satisfied with myself.

We were talking one night about the difference losing weight makes to your life. One particular lady, who was about to reach her goal weight, said to me that in some ways she felt like her innocence had been taken away. When she was an obese person, if she was at a wedding or a party she'd just sit back and watch people, stare at them and admire them living their lives. She'd never participate; instead she watched life from the sidelines. She'd watch people on the dance floor and long to be them. And that's exactly what I used to do.

Now she is out there on the dance floor, too. I suggested to her that losing her weight hadn't taken her innocence away, it had given her life. Life isn't meant to be a passive experience, spent watching the world go by. Life is too short to sit out, you need to participate. It's okay to get out, have a good time and live life.

When I was obese, my life felt like I was on a remote island, like I was Tom Hanks in the movie *Castaway*. He was stuck alone on an island for a couple of years—well, I lived my whole life on that island. And just like when he came back to civilization in the movie, when I lost my weight, I had to learn about a whole new world.

I appreciate the simplest things now because I'd never had them before.... Small things like keeping up with my two young boys, dancing with my husband or taking in the scenery on a nice, long walk. For years no matter how hard I tried I wasn't satisfied with my life because I wasn't satisfied with myself. I'd been stuck on Fat Island and I couldn't get off! My life was constantly about wishing, hoping and praying: wishing I would be slim, hoping I would be pretty, praying people wouldn't laugh at me. Life is still so new for me in so many ways, and I'm learning to live every day. I don't feel like I've lost my innocence; rather, I feel like I've finally joined the world. I've found life and I appreciate every single part of it.

I honestly believe that your weaknesses can make you stronger. If I hadn't been through what I've been through, if I hadn't hit rock bottom and had to climb back up, I wouldn't be the person I am today. I had to fight to gain the life I have, and overcoming the tough times has made me love the challenges life throws my way.

The truth is, feeling good about yourself isn't based on a number on a scale or the label on your dress. Everybody should be content when they look in the mirror, no matter what size they are. I know you are reading this book because you want to lose weight, because you feel trapped in your body and your life. But the pounds are just part of the battle, and if you don't look deep inside yourself and learn to love who you are, you won't be happy at any size.

I also believe that not everyone's goal weight needs to be the same. Your goal should be to lose weight so that you feel healthy and happy. If you reach the weight you're happy with and you're not a size 6, don't worry! As long as you're happy within, that's all that counts.

I often questioned God and myself throughout my life, asking over and over again, "Why is this happening to me?" I believe that we are all born with a particular destiny. My destiny is to use my story to help as many people as I can. My goal is to help others suffering in silence the way I was, to inspire people to create the life they've always dreamed of and to spread the message that you really *can* achieve anything you set your mind to. I also believe that things often happen for a reason—as you embark on the diet and exercise plan on the following pages, always remember that no matter how bad things may get, you can always find sunlight at the end of your journey. We'll do it together.

"Now I love living life."

Maree

Starting Weight: **256** pounds

Current Weight: **192** pounds

64 POUNDS LOST!

I believed I was destined to be overweight all of my life, until I saw an ad for Karen's support group in the local paper. I never mustered the courage to go until my daughter agreed to come with me. The key to my success is controlling my portion sizes and doing some exercise every day. I've learned from Karen that I don't have to run a marathon every day, I just have to move. Like Karen did, I began by walking just for a few minutes each day, then I extended it to laps around my neighborhood and sometimes I've walked up to seven and a half miles a day! I really can't believe how much my life has changed since losing my weight. I look in the mirror and I feel really good. I was never a sociable person—I was too uncomfortable about the way I looked and I was depressed about my size—but now I love getting out and living my life. The Clothesline Diet is the best thing I've ever done.

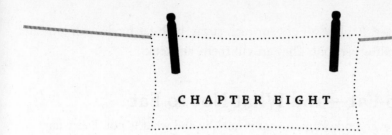

CHAPTER EIGHT

Food, Glorious Food:

Have Your (Low-Fat) Cake and Eat It, Too!

I HAVE ONE VERY STRONG BELIEF ABOUT FOOD AND THAT IS that the more you deprive yourself, the more you crave something and the harder it is to resist. So don't deprive yourself—how easy is that? I could not go through another diet starving myself, I just couldn't. And with my plan, you don't have to.

I could not go through another diet starving myself, I just couldn't. And with my plan, you don't have to.

I also believe that many other diets don't work because they don't teach you how to maintain your weight when you finish dieting. They cut your food down while you are dieting, but when you stop dieting and go back to a "normal" eating plan you put your weight back on. That's why I taught myself to maintain my weight even as I was dieting by following a ten-week cycle: dieting for eight weeks and maintaining for two. During each two-week maintenance period, I had to teach myself how much I could eat before I gained weight—and it worked.

In the following pages, I give you everything you need to follow the Clothesline Diet. As you'll see, it is quite simple and there are hardly any "rules" to follow! All you have to do is think differently about what you eat and how you prepare your food. And I have one simple guideline: replace,

replace, replace. Replace all of your high-sugar, high-fat foods with low-fat, low-sugar healthy versions. They are out there, just look.

What to Eat—and What Not to Eat

Deep down, everybody knows what is healthy and what is not. Every day on TV, in magazines and on billboards, we are bombarded with messages about which foods we should eat and which we should avoid. For the Clothesline Diet, listen to your intuition about what is healthy: foods that are low in fat, low in calories, low in carbohydrates, high in fiber and low in sugar.

The Clothesline Diet is quite simple—and there are hardly any "rules" to follow.

Even though I weighed 300 pounds, I still knew in my heart what was healthy and what wasn't, but the knowledge was useless until I made the decision to use it to change my life. To finally lose weight, I stopped ignoring what I knew and I embraced it. By putting that knowledge into practice, my life changed. I started the diet by quite simply using my own basic knowledge, my eyes and my taste buds.

The key to using my knowledge was to read food labels and understand what I was eating. It's important when you start out to take the time to read labels on packaging because food advertising can be misleading.

It is as simple as that: if it looks bad, it probably is.

Just because an item is low in fat, or low calorie, doesn't mean it's low in sugar, carbs or salt. I always searched for healthier versions of the foods we were already eating—that's important. If I felt like I was starving or depriving myself, it wouldn't have worked. And if my family thought they were missing out, I wouldn't have had their support. Look for healthy choices—they're all around you.

I took a very simple approach to my diet. Just by glancing at packages I could tell if food was bad. For example, chocolate cookies, sugarcoated cereals, different types of spreads, cakes, jelly, salty peanuts, potato chips, peanut butter all had to go. And you know it is as simple as that: if it looks bad, it probably is.

I knew I had to educate myself about fat content and calories because I needed to know how much to burn during exercise. I knew that it would take approximately twenty minutes to burn 110 calories. So when I went to the supermarket, I looked at the package labels, read the calorie content and calculated how much I would have to exercise to burn off that product. It became easy to understand that the fewer the calories, the less I would have to burn in exercise. This way, when I exercised, I would burn my existing fat, rather than the fat from the food that I just ate. How easy is that!

The simplest way to measure what and how much you should be eating is to get yourself a dinner plate or bowl smaller than the one you currently use, and use this bowl for all meals. You will instantly cut down the size of your portions and I bet you'll hardly notice.

Here's my guide, based on what I ate for the main food groups:

Fruits and Vegetables

Eat as much fresh food as possible, particularly fruits and vegetables but remember that some fruits, such as bananas, mangos, pineapple and grapes, can be high in natural sugar. I limited myself to two bananas a week, but I'd still rather you reach for a bowl of grapes than a block of chocolate! As a general guide, too, I ate less white food, such as potatoes and cauliflower, because these are high in carbohydrates. I still ate them, I just cut down the serving size, but I tried to have as wide a variety of colors on my plate as possible.

Natural foods were always my first choice as side dishes. For example, I ate lots of green vegetables and other vegetables that are low in sugar like carrots and peppers, but I limited corn and peas because these are higher in carbohydrates. A mixed salad makes a great alternative to steamed vegetables.

Fat

There were times that my weight loss slowed and at first I couldn't understand why, but when I looked deeper, I found that some of the products I was buying were high in saturated fat. I'd read that saturated fat was bad for you. So when looking at the labels on the packages of products that I would buy, I would now also look at the fat content and see how high in grams the saturated fat was. When I stuck to products that were low in saturated fat, I found that my weight-loss rate would increase again.

Carbohydrates

I have an easy way to tell if something is a carbohydrate—a carbohydrate is "anything white." For example, pasta, bread, potatoes, rice, crackers, cauliflower and peanuts. Don't forget that there are hidden carbs in some foods such as peas, corn and pumpkin. So just limit all white foods and keep in mind that carbs are the hardest thing to burn off—your body loves to store them as fat.

I still ate carbohydrates regularly and I didn't restrict myself to certain times of the day; however, I cut my portions down. If we had pasta or mashed potatoes for dinner, I just ate smaller portions. (Use an ice-cream scoop to measure your portions—it really helps.)

I stopped having sugar in my tea and coffee and stopped using sugar on my cereals. I also kept away from most sweets and candies that contain lots of sugar, and I relied on the natural sugar in natural products like fruit.

Protein

I was never a big meat eater to start with, but I knew that protein gives you energy, so I chose a different range of meats, which I would balance over a period of time, to make sure that I had meat at least twice per week. I ate mainly beef, pork and chicken, but I stayed away from lamb because there is a lot of fat in it.

Fresh fish is a great source of protein and vitamins, so I made sure that I had fresh fish once a week and canned tuna or salmon for lunches twice a week.

Preparing Your Pantry for the New You

When I decided it was time to lose my weight, the first thing I did was clean out my pantry and my fridge. It felt amazing and it signaled to me that I was really serious about changing my life. But it was also a real eye opener. I had bottles and bottles of soda, cookies in all combinations, drawers of snack food. All of it went in the trash. My first shopping trip to fill my new pantry took me hours. I searched shelves and read every label before it went in my basket. I replaced soda, for example, with sugar-free versions, cookies with low-sugar, low-fat versions. I bought low-fat milk, and 99 percent fat-free cheese. And instead of buying multiple choices (we did not need six bottles of soda!) I bought one. But just because you have low-fat, low-sugar foods doesn't mean you can have twice as much! These are only for small servings every now and then.

Stock up on low-fat healthy snacks like rice crackers and healthy cookies, as well as skim milk, low-fat cheese, low-fat yogurt, low-calorie Jell-O (great to snack on if you have a sugar craving), canned fish (great for lunches) and healthy soups.

Don't go crazy and replace everything with tofu and lettuce leaves—your diet will last less than a day! You need to look at what you currently eat. There's no point in starting an eating plan with foods you're going to dislike. Just ease into it, replace the high-fat, high-sugar food with healthier options and, as you go along, gradually remove them from your diet altogether. And if you can, buy in bulk; the fewer trips you make back to the supermarket the better—the less temptation there is to load your cart with unhealthy food. If you buy in bulk you're also more likely to eat what you've got before you buy something new.

Ease into it, replace the high-fat, high-sugar foods with healthier options.

Cooking the Clothesline Way

Changing my cooking methods was really important to the success of the diet—I really had no choice. I couldn't cook the way I always had and expect to lose weight. I deep-fried a lot of food and really didn't choose healthy options when I was cooking. Through a process of trial and error I found new, better ways of making meals. Some of my approaches may make you raise an eyebrow! But they worked for me and I'm sure if you really put your mind to it, you can find much healthier ways of preparing your food. Here are some of my tips:

- I stopped using any oil when I fried food. Instead, I used water for frying, but only a little at a time, enough to keep the food moist so that it doesn't burn. Don't use too much water, otherwise it becomes stewed. It takes a little longer, but in the end it's worth it.

- I steamed all of my vegetables. Some vegetables, such as cabbage, tasted a little bland when steamed, so I added a small amount of mixed herbs or curry to add flavor.

- I used water when baking beef, chicken and pork. I relied on the natural fats in the meat to mix in the water when cooking. Never add oil; you don't need it.

- When I cooked Bolognese sauce for pasta, I used to place my ground meat in a plastic colander over a bowl and precook it in the microwave. This allowed all of the fat to drain out of the meat and into the bowl underneath. I then rinsed the meat under hot water to get out any remaining fat. Then I added the meat to the sauce and allowed it to simmer slowly. This is a lot of work, so if you don't have a lot of time, just use the natural fat in the meat to cook it. But don't add any extra oil and make sure you buy lean meat.

- If you order any kind of salad at a restaurant, always ask for the dressing on the side so that you can add it to the dish moderately and have control over it.

- When making salad dressing at home, I make it with vinegar and lemon juice. You don't need the oil.

- When cooking a barbecue, squeeze a lot of lemon juice over the meat while cooking, because it helps to reduce the fat. Keep well away from sausages unless you make your own with no fat. You can also make your own burgers from low-fat ground meat. Avoid buying prepared burgers from a shop because they contain too much fat and they taste too oily.

- And last, always take the skin off your chicken. It contains most of the chicken's fat.

Simple Clothesline Rules

Before you get started, there are a few simple guidelines that will help you really shed the pounds. If you follow these you can't go wrong:

- Mix and Match: Vary the meals that you and your family eat, including salads and vegetables as much as possible.

- Control Your Portions: Keep your portions small. Your meat and chicken portions should be no larger than the palm of your hand. To measure mashed potatoes (or any other side that's high in carbohydrates) try using an ice-cream scoop. You don't really need more than one scoop of potato at a meal. Try using a small salad plate or a soup bowl for your meals instead of a dinner plate to encourage portion control.

- Eat a Variety of Vegetables: Vegetables are great for the Clothesline Diet because they are low-fat and nutritious! When using vegetables as part of your meal, choose a variety of different vegetables, especially greens. There is a huge range of vegetables to choose from, so make the most of this.

- Eat a Variety of Salads: There is a large range of lettuces you can use for salads. It all comes down to personal choice. Don't limit yourself just to garden salads. There are bean salads, potato salads, coleslaw, rice salads, seafood salads and pasta salads that all make a filling meal or a satisfying side dish. But a word of advice: don't buy ready-made salads, which can be high in fat. Instead, make your own, using low-fat dressings sparingly. Rather than adding fat for flavor, try exploring different seasonings to keep the meal healthy, but still tasty.

- Drink Up: Try to have eight glasses of water per day. It may sound like a lot, but if you break it up throughout the day, it's as easy as can be! I started off with the following: One glass midmorning, three glasses just before lunch, one glass at afternoon snack time and three glasses just before dinner. If this routine doesn't suit you, try two glasses midmorning, two glasses at lunchtime, two glasses in the afternoon and two glasses before dinner—or another combination that works for you. If you absolutely cannot bear the taste of plain water, try mixing low-calorie water flavoring or add a splash of fresh lemon or orange juice into your water jug. This gives the water a bit more taste.

- Eat Five or Six Times a Day: When you feel deprived or hungry, you are more vulnerable to reaching for fattening foods to satisfy cravings. Instead, you should eat three solid meals a day—breakfast, lunch and dinner—along with two to three snacks to ward off hunger and cravings. I suggest having a light midmorning snack and an afternoon snack, as well as one after dinner.

The Ten-Week Cycle

Following the ten-week cycle is important because it will keep you from gaining weight back after all your hard work. Follow my diet plan for eight weeks, then for two weeks try to maintain your weight, allowing yourself treats and foods that you don't eat while trying to lose weight, like a slice of cheesecake. Weigh yourself at the end of eight weeks, then again after two weeks of maintaining. If you put on weight, you know you need to watch your portions during your next maintaining period. If your weight stays the same, you're on the right track.

During the two-week maintenance period, walk only three times each week and drink only five glasses of water a day. Still eat healthily as much as possible. If you are craving food with higher fat content, have something small. For example, try having only a small piece of chocolate, or half a slice of cheesecake, or half a slice of chocolate cake, or two small slices of pizza or a packet of chips, but of course not all in the one sitting! At the end of your two weeks of maintaining, weigh yourself and see if you have gained at all. If you have, don't let it stress you—just acknowledge you have had too much fat and sugar and too many calories during those two weeks. This is the time you will

Once you've reached your goal weight, maintaining will become an everyday part of life for you. It won't be hard at all.

learn how much fat and sugar your body can have before you start gaining weight. If you have still lost some weight, this is a bonus and shows your body has adapted to the weight-loss cycle. If your weight has stayed the same for the two weeks, you are maintaining perfectly.

While you're dieting, you're giving your body a chance to burn the fat it has been storing for years. This is why you need to limit your fat intake. When you're maintaining your weight, you need to control the amount of junk food you consume to allow your body to keep burning the fats in that food. When you reach your goal, you will still need to control the amount of junk food you eat, because if you don't, you will put on weight again.

Once the two weeks of maintaining are over, go back to dieting for another eight weeks. Keep repeating that routine until you hit your goal weight. Once you've reached your goal weight, maintaining will become an everyday part of life for you. Your body will be used to it and it won't be hard at all!

My Super Easy, Seven-Day Diet Plan

This is the diet plan I followed during the eight weeks of every ten-week cycle.

It is the exact diet plan I used to lose my weight, mouthful by mouthful. Use this as a guide to create your own personal diet from the choices I offer in the next section:

Monday

Breakfast	High-fiber, low-fat cereal with skim milk, cup of tea with low-fat milk and no sugar
Midmorning Snack	One piece of fruit, cup of tea
Lunch	Two or three glasses of water. Low-fat soup, two to four plain low-fat crackers topped with tomato, cucumber or low-fat cheese
Afternoon Snack	One small container of low-fat yogurt
Dinner	Two or three glasses of water. Steamed skinless chicken breast and steamed vegetables (as many as you can eat)
After-dinner Snack	Cup of tea, bowl of fresh fruit salad

Tuesday

Breakfast	Two pieces of whole-grain toast with light cream cheese spread, cup of tea
Midmorning Snack	Piece of fruit, cup of tea
Lunch	Two or three glasses of water. Whole-wheat pita bread wrap with tuna, lettuce, cucumber, celery and tomato
Afternoon Snack	One small tub of low-fat yogurt
Dinner	Two or three glasses of water. Small bowl of pasta with low-fat meat sauce
After-dinner Snack	Cup of tea, two or three crackers with light cream cheese spread or low-fat peanut butter

Wednesday

Breakfast	Low-fat cereal of your choice with skim milk, cup of coffee with low-fat milk and no sugar
Midmorning Snack	Small bowl of fruit salad, cup of tea
Lunch	Two or three glasses of water. Big bowl of fresh fruit salad, or low-fat soup
Afternoon Snack	Banana
Dinner	Two or three glasses of water. Grilled fish with rice and steamed vegetables of your choice
After-dinner Snack	Two or three crackers with jelly

Thursday

Breakfast	Two pieces of whole-grain toast with low-fat spread, cup of coffee
Midmorning Snack	Piece of fruit, cup of tea
Lunch	Two or three glasses of water. Two hard-boiled eggs on crackers or rice cakes with low-fat mayonnaise
Afternoon Snack	Small container of low-fat yogurt
Dinner	Two or three glasses of water. Macaroni and cheese, in a very small portion (using low-fat ingredients). Large green salad with lettuce, tomato, cucumber, low-fat cheese
After-dinner Snack	Small bowl of cereal

Friday

Breakfast	Two high-fiber cereal bars with skim milk, cup of tea
Midmorning Snack	Piece of fruit of your choice, cup of tea
Lunch	Two or three glasses of water. Tuna sandwich with salad
Afternoon Snack	Low-fat muesli bar
Dinner	Two or three glasses of water. Chicken stir-fry with vegetables and rice
After-dinner Snack	Two or three crackers with light cream cheese spread

Saturday

Breakfast	Two pieces of soy-and-flaxseed toast with light cream cheese or low-fat peanut butter, cup of tea
Midmorning Snack	Piece of fruit of your choice, cup of tea
Lunch	Two or three glasses of water. Two rice cakes topped with tuna and salad
Afternoon Snack	Piece of fruit of your choice or a small container of yogurt
Dinner	Two or three glasses of water. Whole-wheat pita bread with two hard-boiled eggs, tuna, carrot, celery, lettuce, low-fat cheese
After-dinner Snack	Fresh fruit salad

Sunday

Breakfast	Two pieces of soy-and-flaxseed toast with low-fat cream cheese or low-fat peanut butter, cup of tea
Midmorning Snack	Piece of fruit or small bowl of fresh fruit salad, cup of tea
Lunch	Two or three glasses of water. Roast chicken or beef, with roast potatoes and pumpkin, steamed vegetables of your choice
Dinner	Two or three glasses of water. Sandwich made from lunch leftovers, less the potatoes (I never eat them twice in one day). Add lots of green leafy salad and tomatoes
After-dinner Snack	Fresh fruit salad

A note on portion sizes

- Always consider your portion sizes and keep them within reasonable limits. For example, just because all the food on the diet plan is low in fat doesn't mean you can increase the amount you eat. Use common sense in controlling your meal sizes.

- Don't try to reduce from dinner-plate-sized portions to side-plate-sized ones immediately. Work down to three-quarters of a dinner plate first. After two to four weeks, try reducing to a side plate. This will allow time for your stomach to shrink. The side plate will eventually fill you up; just have patience and trust me. You also need to have your two or three glasses of water, five to ten minutes before your meal to keep you hydrated and fill you up.

Design Your Own Seven-Day Diet Plan

Now that you've seen mine, you can design your own seven-day diet plan. Below is a list of various meal options, covering breakfast, lunch, dinner and snacks. Mix, match or add to this plan, making sure that the meals you prepare are always healthy. I've included a large variety of menus so you don't get bored. Make sure that you don't have more than one portion at each meal—no seconds or thirds. Replace seconds and thirds with more vegetables, salad or fruit. For each meal, choose one of the following options:

Breakfast

(tea, coffee or one glass of low-sugar juice is allowed with any meal)

- Two slices of whole-grain/low-fat bread toasted with light cheese spread or low-sugar jelly

- Two high-fiber cereal bars with low-fat milk

- One slice of toast using low-fat/high-fiber bread, with low-fat spread of your choice and one high-fiber cereal bar with low-fat milk

- Small bowl of low-fat, low-sugar cereal with low-fat milk

- Two low-fat English muffins with low-fat spread

- One poached egg with one or two slices of low-fat toast

- One slice of raisin toast with a small bowl of any low-fat cereal

- Two slices of raisin toast with tea, coffee or juice

Breakfast Tips

- Add choices to the list as you wish but ensure that any choice is low in fat.

- Remember you can mix and match the above depending on what suits you; it's important you don't get bored eating the same foods.

- Don't have two slices of bread for breakfast and again for lunch or dinner. Limit your bread intake to eight slices per week.

- You don't need to have two slices of toast and a bowl of cereal. Choose only one of each for each sitting.

Morning Snack

Your choice of one of the following:

- Any piece of fruit (see "Tips" about limiting number of bananas)

- Tea or coffee with two low-fat, low-sugar cookies

- Small container of low-fat yogurt

- Tea or coffee with one small low-fat muffin
- Bowl of mixed fruit
- Low-fat muesli bar

Midmorning Snack Tips

- Limit bananas to two per week. They are high in sugar and protein.
- Always have one glass of water before you have your midmorning snack.
- Try not to replace your midmorning snack with your lunch. This will cause you to deviate from your routine.
- If you are still hungry after your midmorning snack, have extra fruit.

Lunch

(Always have three glasses of water, five to ten minutes before eating)

- A cup of low-fat soup with four low-fat crackers, tomatoes and cucumber
- Low-fat, three-minute rice meal
- Low-fat, two-minute instant noodles bowl (such as instant Thai noodles)
- Half a whole-grain pita bread with low-fat mayonnaise, tuna packed in springwater, lettuce and tomatoes
- Salad of your choice—chicken, tuna, egg, vegetarian—sandwich on low-fat bread
- Large fruit salad
- 99 percent fat-free cup of soup with a small bowl of fruit salad
- Two hard-boiled eggs with low-fat crackers and low-fat mayonnaise. You can use low-fat bread if you wish, instead of crackers, to allow you to have it as a sandwich.
- Ham and lettuce sandwich using low-fat bread and no butter. Use light cheese spread, low-fat mayonnaise or mustard pickles instead.
- Cold grilled chicken on a whole-grain roll with or without lettuce. You can add low-fat mayonnaise.
- A container of low-fat yogurt and a bowl of fruit

- Here is one of my Sunday lunch favorites: one roast potato, two pieces of squash with a medium slice of beef, or a piece of skinless chicken with heaps of vegetables—peas, carrots, beans, broccoli, corn—whatever your family prefers. I suggest you steam the lighter vegetables but roast the pumpkin and potato in water (not oil). Have with one slice of low-fat bread. Bake roasts in water, not oil.

- Six low-fat crackers served with ricotta or cottage cheese and tomatoes

Lunch Tips

- Mix and match or add alternatives to the list, if you wish, provided new alternatives are low-fat items.

- When going shopping look carefully because there are so many kinds of low-fat crackers that are fantastic for lunches.

- If you happen to be out at lunchtime, look for healthy food options like those in this menu.

- All lunch meals can be served with orange juice, coffee or tea.

- If you have the time after eating, a twenty-minute walk will keep your metabolism going.

Afternoon Snack
(One glass of water before eating)

- One low-fat muesli bar

- One health bar, such as a low-fat cereal bar

- A banana

- A bowl of fruit salad served with low-fat yogurt cup

- A small bowl of low-sugar Jell-O with a portion of canned fruit

- One chopped carrot with a celery stick and a low-fat dip of your choice

- Six water crackers with slices of low-fat cheese

- Stewed apples with or without low-fat pudding

- Two oranges cut into slices

Afternoon Snack Tips

- We often get hungry between 3:00 and 5:00 p.m. while preparing for dinner. Make up a bowl of fruit salad and have a fork handy so you can pick at the salad while cooking.

- You could also have a few water crackers or even a handful of dried fruits with raw mixed nuts (not roasted in oil).

- Remember not to eat too much at this time, because dinner is not far away.

Dinner
(Always have three glasses of water, five to ten minutes before your meal)

- Steamed or boiled skinless chicken fillets, one hard-boiled egg, moderate serving of steamed vegetables or salad

- One piece of pork chop baked in water, one cup of cooked pasta, served with vegetables

- Fried rice (fried in water) mixed with stir-fry of your choice. Try looking for low-fat stir-fries to try. This can also be served with steamed vegetables.

- Grilled fish with salad

- Portion of skinless chicken, served with a small portion of steamed potato and vegetables. I buy chicken schnitzel without bread crumbs from the butcher. I like the schnitzel because it's a thinner chicken portion and cooks quickly. But you could use any skinless chicken fillet.

- Pita bread with low-fat mayonnaise, tuna and salad

- Chicken or beef stir-fry

- Bread-plate-sized serving of macaroni and cheese, baked rice or spaghetti, served with low-fat sauces

- Omelet, using two eggs, tomatoes, ham; low-fat cheese on a sandwich using low-fat bread

- Two medium-sized beef hamburgers cooked using low-fat ground beef, one medium-sized boiled potato and one ear of corn. If you don't feel like hamburgers, you can try turkey burgers, or tuna or chicken patties.

- Homemade pizza using pita bread bases and all the healthy ingredients you can think of sprinkled on top. You can mix and match the toppings to your taste. Limit how much cheese you use and make sure it's low-fat.

- Homemade minestrone, chicken or pumpkin soup—be sure to limit the quantity of potato in any soup

- Grilled T-bone steak served with a gravy sauce, coleslaw mixed with low-fat mayonnaise and a medium-sized baked potato filled with a light stuffing of your choice (a tomato can be substituted for the potato)

Dinner Tips

- I'm sure I'm not the only one who looks forward to dinnertime. Remember that it is the last main meal of the day and usually we tend to become lazy after it. I recommend getting out for even a ten-minute walk after dinner. You can make it a family outing. It is a great idea, especially during daylight savings time, and will give your metabolism a chance to keep burning excess fat.

Evening Snack

- A small bowl of fruit salad, or a piece of fruit

- A small bowl of low-fat pretzels

- A cup of tea or coffee with two low-fat cookies

- Four water crackers with low-fat cheese or peanut butter

- A cup of low-fat hot chocolate with a small low-fat muffin

- A small bowl of low-fat cereal with low-fat milk

- A small container of low-fat yogurt

Evening Snack Tips

- If you can live without an evening snack, then do so. I know it's easier said than done, but remember, this is the last food that you will consume before going to bed, so you don't have many hours left in the day to burn it off! Have the smallest portion possible. One of my favorite evening snacks was a cup of low-cal hot chocolate without milk.

Tips for Getting Started

To start, design your own diet plan for the week, or use mine just to get you started. Once you have decided on a diet plan, start weighing yourself to monitor your results. If the scales are showing you're 220 pounds, say, don't get stressed—you're about to start the greatest journey of your life. Whisper these magic words: "Not for long!"

You're about to start the greatest journey of your life.

Now you're ready. Follow your eight-week plan strictly. Keep weighing yourself once a week to encourage yourself along the way, but absolutely no more than once a week; don't let the scales control you. Quite often your weight fluctuates from day to day depending on fluid and it can be really depressing and discouraging if you feel your weight isn't budging. It's really important that you don't spend every day standing on scales. Pick one day to weigh yourself once a week and that is all. Live a normal life and don't let dieting take it over. If you treat your diet plan as a life change, it actually will become part of your everyday life.

Live a normal life and don't let dieting take it over.

Always remember to limit portion sizes, have your six to eight glasses of water a day. You'll also want to exercise for at least twenty minutes, five days a week—see the next chapter for more details At the end of the eighth week, record your weight. I anticipate you should have lost approximately ten to twenty pounds. For the following two weeks, concentrate on maintaining your weight.

> ## "When I see a big person now, I want to tell them their life can be so different."

Kerry

Starting Weight: **216** pounds

Current Weight: **128** pounds

88 POUNDS LOST!

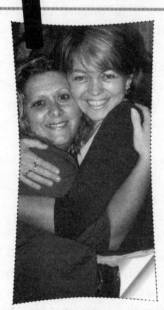

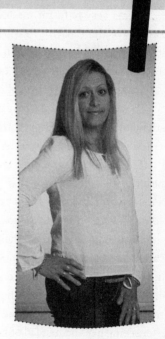

On left

There was no better way to celebrate turning forty than to show off a new body! Losing weight was one of the biggest hurdles I have ever overcome and achieving it changed my life forever. By losing the weight I'd given myself the best birthday present ever—the gift of life.

My weight, and my life for that matter, had been spiraling out of control for a long time. I have four beautiful children, but life hasn't been easy. I'd been steadily getting fatter for about twenty years. I put on weight after each of my four pregnancies. I put on weight when I was depressed, I put on weight when I was bored. I put on weight for just about every reason, but I never really seemed to take it off. I'd lose a few pounds, then gain a few more.

I've had a lot of ups and downs in my life, but my life really spiraled out of control when I put my disabled daughter into foster care. She was seven years old and needed twenty-four-hour care, and I was a single mother with two children—and I am deaf. I just couldn't provide her with the attention she needed. Giving away Tamara was a major turning point in my life. It was the beginning of the downfall, really. I plunged into a very deep depression. That's when I really put on weight. I basically sat on the couch and ate anything around me and the weight packed on. I didn't know what else to do. Food seemed to soothe the hurt I was feeling inside as well as give me something to do to pass the time.

It was very hard for me to go to commercial diet centers—they didn't really have the capacity to cope with deaf people. To be honest I had very little motivation to lose weight anyway, and that made my depression worse because I hated myself for not being motivated to lose weight!

I didn't want to go through the rest of my life like that.

So when I picked up a magazine a few weeks later and read Karen's story, I thought it was fate. Everything about it hit me right in the heart. It really struck a chord with me, and she looked fantastic after losing her weight.

This might sound a little crazy, but I knew I had to meet her. Karen gave me a tiny little bit of hope that I might just be able to do what she had. I read her story over and over again and said to my son Wayne, "You must call this woman for me." She told me to come to her meeting and I did.

Wayne came with me to help translate, which really put my mind at ease. Karen explained what had happened in her life and how she'd lost her weight, and it was very emotional. I cried and cried. I could understand everything she'd been through and for the first time in my life, I didn't feel alone. She made such sense and mirrored what was going on in my life. I'd get home after seeing her and instead of heading for the couch, I'd walk for an hour! My motivation was sky-high and I felt so good.

In the beginning I did exactly what Karen did and I walked around my backyard because I was too embarrassed to walk on the street. Then when I felt brave, I'd walk around the block.

It wasn't long before I could actually see I was losing weight and my confidence was growing and growing. Now I walk every day—I can't stand it if I don't.

Karen talked me through what I should and shouldn't have, and what to replace my meals with so I wasn't missing out. I never really felt like I was on a diet because I still ate the food I loved, I just replaced unhealthy ingredients with low-fat, low-sugar options.

Sixteen months after I met Karen I'd reached my goal weight. I was 128 pounds and I felt fabulous. When I think that it took twenty years for my life to unravel, and just sixteen months to turn it around, I wish I'd met Karen years ago!

Whenever I see a big person now I desperately want to tell them that their life can be so different.

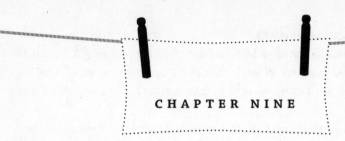

CHAPTER NINE

Step to It:
Shed Those Pounds Without Ever Going to the Gym

YOU DON'T HAVE TO BE AN ACTIVE PERSON TO EXERCISE, AND you don't have to be fit to start walking. Always keep in mind how I started exercising. I thought I was way too big to exercise. I struggled to walk to my mailbox—really, it's true!—so going out for a walk was not happening. No way!

And as for going to the gym—you've got to be kidding. I tried gyms years ago, but I hated having people who had never had a weight problem tell me what to do. And even worse—the equipment. Oh, my God! I couldn't sit on an exercise bike because the seat disappeared under my bum. I couldn't fit my bottom cheeks on an exercise bike and the fat used to hang over the sides. How embarrassing. And most normal treadmills couldn't hold my weight, so that ruled them out. And what's with gyms having so many mirrors? The reason most people are there is because they are overweight. Who wants to look at themselves at their worst? It's just a reminder of how much work you have to do!

I knew I had to do some exercise because my weight wasn't going to come off otherwise, but I had to start slowly and I had to feel comfortable about it. That's why I chose to walk around the clothesline in my backyard. I could go at my own pace, no one could see me and I felt perfectly comfortable. I started walking for five minutes a day, just five minutes because that was all I could do. And honestly, on that first day I felt like I was having a heart attack. My heart was pounding, I was sweating and I had to hold on to the line to keep myself up, but I did it. And after that first day it got easier and easier. It may sound funny, but my clothesline became my best friend.

After that first day it got easier and easier. It may sound funny, but my clothesline became my best friend.

As each day went by, I added one minute to my walk and kept on adding a minute a day, until I reached twenty minutes a day. I stuck to this on my ten-week plan. Walking gave me the chance to get in touch with my inner spirit and think about my goals and achievements. It made me believe in myself more and more each day. Who knows? This could happen to you—but you have to give yourself the chance. It all comes back to believing in yourself and enjoying the process of getting healthy.

Exercise Outside of the Box

There are loads of fantastic activities you can do to help you lose weight, so don't just think of exercise as going to a gym for an hour or going for a walk: think outside the box. Do whatever strikes your fancy. Maybe you like bike riding with your kids, maybe you like aerobics, line dancing, yoga, golf? It's really up to you, as long as you do something every day. I chose walking, pure and simple.

And have a look around you. Everyone can find somewhere to start exercising at home. Maybe you have stairs or a driveway to walk up and down. One Clothesline dieter who lived in the Outback started walking a few kilometers along the fence to her mailbox every day, instead of driving to it as she always had; one lady walked laps of the hallway in her suburban house. Have a look for exercise DVDs, too. There are so many around and some very good ones out there that can help you get moving in the privacy of your own home. Find your own "clothesline."

Take It One Step at a Time

I was 300 pounds when I began my daily walks. I could barely take a step, but I just put one foot in front of the other and kept going, one step at a time. I love my walks now and I still walk every day just to clear my head. But boy, it was hard to begin with.

By the time I'd lost about 45 pounds, I had added some sit-ups to my routine. But again, I started slowly: five one day, six the next. Don't expect that you will walk out the front door and run a marathon the first time you exercise. Take it slowly. Go at the pace you are comfortable with and enjoy the exercise you do. It shouldn't be a chore. Remember, though, do exercise every day; make it a part of your routine.

You're the one who has to want this, and you have to want it in your heart, not just in your mind.

I believe that if you need to lose 10 pounds or 100 pounds, you still need to have the same inspiration, motivation, self-confidence and belief in yourself. My goal is to help and support you in any way I can. You need to remember that you're the one who has to want this, and you have to want it in your heart, not just in your mind. You have to make it happen for yourself. Losing weight is an enormous battle—every day is a challenge—but as each day goes by, it does get easier. Always remember that if somebody like me can do it, anybody can.

Exercise Options

I have put together a number of exercise options that you can mix and match to suit your lifestyle. You can do many types of different kinds of exercise. It's just a matter of finding activities that you enjoy and making time for them in your daily routine. Unfortunately, when most of us think of exercise we automatically think of hard work and hours spent sweating it out at the gym. We never actually stop and think that exercise can be fun. I have included exercises

If somebody like me can do it, anybody can.

that are very easy to follow, are fun and won't eat a hole in your wallet! They are all designed to help you burn up lots of calories without even realizing it. The best part about most of these activities is that they can be done alone or with friends and family.

It doesn't matter what size or shape you are—everyone can do these exercises at their own pace. It's all about getting back to basics, having fun and treating your weight loss as a life change, not just another weekly diet. I follow this approach at my camps and my support groups and we always have a good time—and lose weight, too! Enjoy.

Walking or Power Walking

Now, there's no excuse not to go for a walk. Walking is an activity everyone can do, at any time. Start off walking at a slow pace then gradually work it up to a pace where you feel your heart rate is pumping and you begin to sweat. Use your arms to keep your pace and pick up speed, remembering to keep your arms bent at the elbows. Make sure your back and posture are straight to allow you to breathe properly, and lean forward slightly when walking up hills. Aside from being a fantastic way to lose weight and tone up your body overall, walking offers a chance to clear your mind and focus on your well-being and your goals; it's a terrific total mind and body workout.

> **Tips:** *If you are embarrassed about walking on the streets or in public, do what I did and walk laps in your backyard first until you lose a little weight and build up your confidence and fitness.*

- Point your thumbs forward at all times to help your shoulders stay back; this will also improve your posture. Walk with confidence—you are on a mission!

- When you feel comfortable, increase your activity level by adding a small set of hand weights to your walk.

- Try to carry a water bottle with you, but if it's too uncomfortable, make sure you drink two to three glasses of water as soon as you get home.

- If you are walking on a treadmill, start off slowly. Increase the pace a fraction at a time until you are slightly out of your comfort zone, then hold that pace.

Jogging

There is no point in even attempting to jog until you are well into your journey and walking at a fast pace. If you feel that walking is no longer doing enough for you and your body is giving you signs it wants to increase the pace, then go for it, but start slowly and build up your confidence. If you feel you are ready to give jogging a go, start building yourself up by slowly jogging in short bursts. Try jogging across each street you come to or jogging for ten to fifteen seconds every two minutes.

Swimming

Swimming laps either up and down the length of the pool or across the width of the pool is a fantastic form of exercise and can be really beneficial for people wanting to lose weight. It is especially effective for larger people who have issues with legs and lower back pain. Swimming takes away the impact on your joints and allows you to exercise freely. Likewise, water aerobics is a terrific form of low-impact exercise that can really benefit weight loss.

Backyard Basketball

You don't have to be a professional basketball player to reap the benefits of shooting a few hoops. All you need is a basic knowledge of the game. And if you don't know the rules, make them up as you go along! The concept is simple: score points by getting the ball in the hoop. If you don't have a basketball hoop in your backyard, head to the nearest school as most have a basketball hoop and court set up. You can play by yourself (great for toning your arms) or with two or more people.

Backyard Volleyball

Backyard volleyball is so simple. All you have to do is keep the ball off the ground and tap it over the net. Points are scored when either team lets the ball hit the ground. This can be played with as few as two players on each side and can be great fun. I play this with Jason and our boys on the beach or in the park and it gives you a great overall body workout. It is especially good for toning up flabby arms!

Tip: *If you don't have a net, just use a piece of rope.*

Climbing Steps

Walking up and down steps or sidewalk curbs is an excellent way to work your legs, thighs and hips anytime, day or night, and all of us have at least a set of steps or a curb nearby. It sounds like a simple exercise and it is, but you can always spice it up a bit. For instance, as you step up with one foot, lift your other leg up high, aiming to get your knee as close to your chest as possible, then return to start. Do eight to ten repetitions on each side. If you don't have any steps in your house, use the curbs outside or buy a small plastic step from the local hardware store. They cost only a few dollars and are a great exercise tool.

Three-Legged Races

Remember how much fun this was as a child? Well, I can safely say you laugh as much, if not more so, doing this as an adult. We compete in three-legged races at my camps, and boy do we laugh. It's a really fun exercise and helps you develop a good rhythm. It also offers a terrific workout for legs, waist and hips, along with a few good belly laughs. Be sure to use a wide strap or band to tie around the ankles to avoid any bruising, and keep a good grip on your partner's waist.

Bike Riding

Now, everyone can ride a bike—no excuses! If a child can do it, you can! Even if it's been a while since you dusted off the old bike, don't despair, it only takes a few minutes to quickly remember exactly what you're doing. Bike riding is similar to walking in that you can do it on your own and it gives you time to focus on yourself and reflect on your journey and your goals. There's nothing better than a great bike ride in the fresh air to lift your spirits and make you feel really good about yourself. Like any other exercise, start off slowly until you build up your confidence, just go up and down the driveway or around the block until you get your bike legs, then hit the nearest park or bike path and enjoy!

An exercise bike is also a terrific weight-loss tool, with the added advantage that if you have one you can do it in the privacy of your own home at any time. Get yourself into a routine of riding the exercise bike for twenty to thirty minutes three times a week. Flick on your favorite TV show and cycle slowly while you're watching it—even though you're watching television, you're still burning fat.

Circuits

Exercise circuits are easy to organize and can combine lots of fun activities; this is a great family exercise. This list is an example of the circuits I coordinate at our camps and support groups. You can use one of mine or create your own.

Place each activity station about 3–4 yards apart. On the blow of a whistle (or your own stopwatch) carry out each activity for two minutes before moving to the next exercise. This can be done on your own or in a group. By the time everyone gets back to their original station, you will have done around twenty solid minutes of heart-pumping work.

1. **Skipping rope**
2. **Small Arm Weights:** using small weights, lift your arms up and down slowly.
3. **Punching Pads:** bend into a squat position, punching your arms out as you return to stance. With each squat and return to position, punch your arms out hard, following a bend and punch motion.
4. **Hula-Hoops:** place six hoops down on the ground in pairs and in a line and run through the hoops, placing a foot inside each one as you go. Run as fast as you can.
5. **Basketball:** bounce the ball in figure eights around your legs.
6. **Squats:** Write *squats* on a piece of cardboard and place it on the ground in front of you. With your hands on your hips, squat up and down as slowly as you can. Get as low to the floor and the card as possible.

Give each activity as much effort as possible, you will use different muscle groups with each one, so the workout is quite comprehensive. Mix and match activities; just about any exercise can be included in a circuit.

Ball Work

These are a few short activities you can do anywhere providing you have a ball—a basketball is ideal.

- Throw the ball up in the air and clap twice before you catch it
- Holding the ball out in front of you, your arms stretched out straight, carry out a series of ten slow full squats
- Bounce the ball through your legs in figure eights
- Holding the ball at your chest, twist at the waist, ensuring your hips are straight

Do each of these activities for two minutes, before moving on to the next one.

Dancing

I am definitely making up for lost time here, but I love dancing and I will dance anywhere. For so many years I refused to get anywhere near the dance floor—in fact I wished it would open up and swallow me, I was so embarrassed by my size. Now you can't keep me away from it! I have a huge range of music at home and a big stereo system and I dance and sing whenever I get the chance. Sometimes Jason and the boys will run across the road to the park to get away from my loud singing and dancing! You don't have to be a disco freak or a superstar dancer. Just play your favorite music and let your body move to the beat. You can also learn some of the more popular party dances or line dances. It doesn't matter how you move, as long as you do it.

Aerobics Videos

There are so many good aerobics videos available these days there really is no excuse not to exercise at home. Choose a video that suits your level of fitness and exercise to your heart's content. Aerobics videos are also fun for the kids and they love to join in, so why not do this as a fun after-school activity for everyone.

Hallway or Stairway Walking

I walked around the clothesline in my backyard to lose weight. Many people think this is strange, and I often get raised eyebrows when I tell people about it, but it worked! If you feel uncomfortable walking in public, why not walk up and down your hallway, staircase or around your backyard. It's a good way to get your body moving and you can keep an eye on your baby, the cooking or even the TV. The point is, there really should be no excuse for not exercising, anywhere, anytime. But to be successful, it must be part of your everyday life. Exercising at home is a great way to kick off your journey.

Tips for Success

Always wear properly fitted sports shoes because your legs and feet are your foundation. Start any exercise routine slowly to suit your pace and fitness level, then work your way up to a level that is out of your comfort zone. This can take weeks or months, and remember—*no excuses!*

"My sister inspired me to change my life."

Aaron

Starting Weight: **256** pounds

Current Weight: **198** pounds

67 POUNDS LOST!

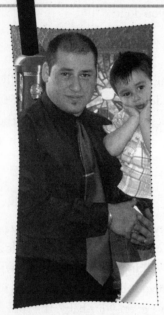
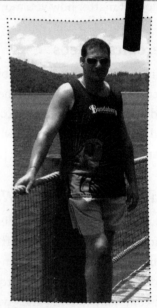

I have lost 67 pounds thanks to the motivation and encouragement that Karen gave me. Karen is my older sister and I've watched her struggle with weight all of her life. I was battling it, too. We have always had a very close bond, and our weight was a shared problem. I was so proud when Karen lost her weight that it prompted me to finally take control of my life, too. I figured that if Karen could do it, I could, too. I hated being overweight; it was hard living life as a big man. My self-esteem was terrible and I didn't like the way I looked. I wasn't living life to the fullest. I was only thirty and really my weight should've been the last thing on my mind, but I was very unhappy.

When Karen started her journey back in 1999, we started it together. There was never a day that she did not encourage me and support me in every way. She taught me my new eating habits and even taught me how to exercise the old-fashioned way. I worked as a cabinetmaker, fitting wardrobes in new houses, Karen taught me to park my van at the front of the houses where I worked and not in the driveways, so I could walk farther. She always suggested power walking or running up and down the stairs when I had to work in two-story houses and I always took her advice. They were simple changes, but they worked.

We would call each other every day to see how we were doing on our journey. I would see her determination and passion and that was the inspiration I needed.

Today I have so much confidence within my life and myself. I love water sports and motorcycle riding, and I am extremely active and always on the go with my two beautiful children. I have now maintained my weight for years and embrace life every single day—and, yes, Karen still is my inspiration.

CHAPTER TEN

Favorite Clothesline Recipes

One of the best things about my diet is the food! I never starved and had so much fun trying new foods and creating new meals for my family. We have new favorites now and I try to create different meals regularly so they don't get bored. Once a month during my support group we have a cooking night, when everyone brings in a new favorite dish for us to try and then we talk about how they took an old recipe and transformed it. It's usually a meal that's an old favorite they've made over in a new, healthy way. So I wanted to include a few basic healthy recipes you can follow. There's a range of delicious starters, entrées, even desserts. Take these recipes and use them as a guide to create your own new favorites.

Vegetable Omelet

SERVES 4

4 eggs, beaten

2 tsp parsley

1 cup vegetable stock

1 tsp curry powder

½ cup chopped carrots

½ cup green beans

½ cup potatoes, cubed

½ cup pumpkin, cubed

½ cup mushroom, diced

½ cup zucchini, diced

½ cup green pepper, diced

½ cup red pepper, diced

1 medium onion, diced

canola oil, to spray

2 tomatoes, sliced

1. Preheat oven to 350°F.

2. Combine eggs with parsley, stock and curry powder.

3. Steam carrots, beans, potatoes and pumpkin until just tender, and add to egg mixture.

4. Fry mushrooms, zucchini, green and red peppers, and onions without oil then add to egg mixture.

5. Lightly spray 1 quart casserole dish with canola oil and pour mixture in.

6. Place sliced tomatoes on top of mixture.

7. Bake at 350°F until omelet is golden brown.

Tip: *You can leave out the potatoes or substitute them for another vegetable.*

Nutrition Information Per Serving: 171 calories, 18g carbs, 9g protein, 4g fiber, 8g fat

Low-Fat Scones

MAKES 18–20 SCONES

4 cups of self-rising flour	1 cup of low-fat cream
1 pinch of salt	1 cup of sugar-free lemonade

1. Preheat oven to 400°F.
2. Mix all ingredients in a large bowl.
3. Knead into a dough and flatten with your palm until about 1 inch thick.
4. Cut out scones and put on to a greased baking sheet.
5. Bake for 9 minutes in a convection oven, or 12 minutes for normal oven, or until golden brown.

   Whip up some low-fat cream with some low-sugar jam and enjoy!

Nutrition Information Per Serving: 125 calories, 21g carbs, 3g protein, 1g fiber, 3g fat

Banana and Rolled-Oat Muffins

MAKES 12 MUFFINS

2 cups self-rising flour

1 tsp ground cinnamon

½ tsp baking soda

1 cup rolled oats

½ cup brown sugar

2 eggs

¾ cup plain low-fat yogurt

¼ cup canola oil

2 bananas, mashed (2 cups)

1. Preheat oven to 400°F. Line a 12-cup muffin pan with paper liners.

2. Sift flour, cinnamon and baking soda into a bowl. Empty the flour husks remaining in the sifter into the bowl along with the oats and brown sugar, and stir to combine.

3. Whisk eggs, yogurt and oil together. Add banana and stir to combine. Pour into dry ingredients and mix together using a wooden spoon until just combined. Mixture may be lumpy and does not have to be evenly mixed.

4. Spoon mixture into cups. Bake for 20 minutes or until golden and cooked through. Cool for 5 minutes before transferring to a wire rack to cool completely.

Nutrition Information Per Serving: 230 calories, 39g carbs, 5g protein, 2g fiber, 6g fat

Baked Onions Stuffed with Pistachios and Dried Cranberries

SERVES 10

10 medium brown onions, unpeeled

2 tbsp extra virgin olive oil

6 oz bacon slices, trimmed of fat and chopped

4 garlic cloves, finely chopped

1 tbsp finely chopped fresh thyme

1 ½ tsp finely grated lemon rind

1 ⅔ cups fresh bread crumbs (made from day-old whole-wheat bread)

½ cup unsalted pistachio kernels, finely chopped

½ cup dried cranberries

1 egg, lightly whisked

Salt & freshly ground black pepper

1. Preheat oven to 400°F. Place whole onions in a large saucepan and cover with cold water. Bring to a boil over high heat. Reduce heat to medium-low and simmer, partly covered, for 15 minutes or until tender. Remove from heat. Drain. Set aside for 20 minutes to cool.

2. Peel the onions. Use a small sharp knife to trim the base and top of each onion, and discard. Use a teaspoon to scoop out the flesh, leaving a ½-inch border. Reserve 1 cup of onion flesh and finely chop. Set aside. Place onion shells on a baking tray.

3. Heat the oil in a large frying pan over medium heat. Add the reserved onion, bacon, garlic, thyme and lemon rind, and cook, stirring, for 5 minutes or until bacon is golden brown. Transfer to a heat-proof bowl and set aside for 5 minutes to cool.

(continued)

4. Add the bread crumbs, pistachios, dried cranberries and egg to the bacon mixture, and stir to combine. Season with salt and pepper. Spoon filling into the onion shells. Bake in preheated oven for 30 minutes or until golden brown and tender.

Nutrition Information Per Serving: 223 calories, 29g carbs, 7g protein, 3g fiber, 9g fat

Cheesy Vegetable Pots

SERVES 4

2 carrots, peeled, diced into small squares

7 oz broccoli, trimmed, cut into small florets

7 oz cauliflower, trimmed, cut into small florets

¼ cup light cream cheese

¼ cup plain flour

2 cups low-fat milk, warmed

1 cup grated low-fat cheddar cheese

1. Place carrots in a shallow microwave-safe dish. Add 2 to 3 tablespoons cold water. Cover and microwave on high for 4 to 5 minutes or until tender. Remove to a bowl. Place broccoli and cauliflower in the dish. Add a little more water if necessary. Cover and microwave on high for 3 to 4 minutes or until tender. Drain well.

2. Preheat oven to 400°F. Divide vegetables between four greased 1½ cup ovenproof dishes. Set aside.

3. Melt cream cheese in a small saucepan over medium heat. Remove pan from heat. Stir in flour. Return to medium heat. Cook, stirring, for 1 to 2 minutes or until mixture forms bubbles. Remove from heat. Slowly add milk, whisking constantly until smooth. Return to heat. Cook, stirring, for 1 to 2 minutes or until sauce comes to a boil and thickens. Reduce heat to low and simmer for 2 minutes or until thickened. Stir in half the cheese.

4. Spoon sauce over vegetables. Sprinkle with remaining cheese. Place dishes on a baking tray. Bake for 15 to 20 minutes or until cheese melts and is golden. Set aside for 5 minutes to cool slightly. Serve.

Nutrition Information Per Serving: 220 calories, 24g carbs, 17g protein, 4g fiber, 7g fat

Curried Lentil and Pumpkin Soup

SERVES 6

1 tbsp olive oil

1 onion, finely chopped

1 clove garlic, crushed

2 tsp Madras curry powder

1 ½ cups dried red lentils

3 ¾ lbs pumpkin, peeled, seeds removed and chopped (you can use butternut squash if you prefer)

5 cups vegetable stock

plain yogurt, to garnish

1. Heat oil in a large heavy-based saucepan over medium heat. Add onion and garlic, cooking for 2 to 3 minutes until soft. Stir in curry powder and cook, stirring, for 30 seconds.

2. Add lentils, pumpkin, and stock. Stir until well combined. Bring to a boil, then reduce heat to medium-low. Cook, partially covered, for about 20 minutes, stirring often until pumpkin is just tender.

3. Serve immediately, topped with a dollop of plain yogurt if desired.

Nutrition Information Per Serving: 320 calories, 51g carbs, 19g protein, 8g fiber, 6g fat

Easy Pork Patties

SERVES 4

10 oz pork fillet

1 egg, beaten

½ cup self-rising flour

1 small cucumber, finely chopped

½ red pepper, finely chopped

3 spring onions, finely chopped

1 tbsp olive oil

1. Grind pork in food processor. In a large bowl, mix pork, egg, self-rising flour, cucumber, pepper and spring onions and blend for 60 seconds.

2. Heat oil in nonstick frying pan and cook teaspoonfuls of mixture over medium heat until golden brown on both sides.

Nutritional Information Per Serving: 196 calories, 16g carbs, 18g protein, 1g fiber, 7g fat

Chicken and Ricotta Fingers

SERVES 4

14 oz lean ground chicken

1 egg

3 ½ oz low-fat ricotta cheese

1 large carrot, finely grated

1 medium onion, finely diced

1 large zucchini, grated

3 tbsp whole-wheat flour

seasoning to taste

1. Place all ingredients into a large bowl and mix well to combine.
2. Shape mixture into small finger-shaped logs and place on a tray lined with wax paper.
3. Place tray in the refrigerator for 30 minutes to set before cooking.
4. Steam fingers in a vegetable steamer over boiling water in batches for 10 minutes or until cooked through.

Nutrition Information Per Serving: 256 calories, 16g carbs, 24g protein, 3g fiber, 11g fat

Mediterranean Style Tuna with Brussels Sprouts

SERVES 4

1 tsp olive oil

½ red pepper, finely sliced into 2-inch-long strips

4–5 shallots, chopped

2 cloves garlic, crushed

2 tbsp pine nuts, dry roasted in pan

9 oz tomatoes, peeled and chopped

1 tsp sugar

13 oz Brussels sprouts, washed well and sliced in halves or quarters

2 tbsp fresh basil, chopped (or 1 tsp dried basil)

21 oz firm fish (for example, tuna, salmon, mackerel or bluefish), chopped into large chunks

cracked black pepper, to taste

10 oz whole-wheat pasta, cooked and drained

1. Heat the oil in a frying pan or wok and stir-fry the peppers, shallots, garlic and pine nuts for 2 to 3 minutes.

2. Add the tomatoes, sugar, sprouts, basil and fish, and cook, covered, for 5 to 7 minutes.

3. Season with the pepper .

   To serve, spoon mixture immediately over cooked pasta.

Nutrition Information Per Serving: 357 calories, 31g carbs, 42g protein, 6g fiber, 8g fat

CROWD-PLEASING LUNCHES AND DINNERS

Spinach and Cheese Meat Loaf

SERVES 6

26 oz 95% lean ground beef

1 onion, chopped

2 eggs

½ cup fresh bread crumbs (multigrain)

1 tbsp teriyaki sauce

3 slices bacon, trimmed of all fat and chopped

1 bunch spinach leaves, washed and chopped (you can also use Swiss chard)

1 cup low-fat grated cheddar cheese

1 tbsp water

1. Preheat oven to 350°F.

2. Process meat and onion in food processor until smooth, add eggs, bread crumbs and teriyaki sauce, then process until combined.

3. Cook bacon in nonstick pan until crisp then remove, drain fat and clean pan. In same pan add spinach and bacon with 1 to 2 tbsp of water. Cover and cook 1 to 2 minutes, cool, then process spinach mixture until smooth.

4. Spread mince mixture from step 2 on a 9 x 11 inch sheet of aluminum foil to about 1 inch thick, spread spinach mixture over mince mixture, then top with cheese. Roll up lengthwise like a swiss roll, and tuck ends under to enclose spinach mixture.

5. Place meat loaf seam side down on a baked dish or in an oblong dish. Bake at 350°F for 50 minutes. To microwave, cook meat loaf on high for about 15 minutes. Not suitable to freeze.

Nutrition Information Per Serving: 368 calories, 12g carbs, 47g protein, 2g fiber, 14g fat

Chicken and Ricotta Pasta Bake

SERVES 4

6 oz uncooked spiral whole-wheat pasta

1 ½ cups coarsely chopped zucchini

1 medium green pepper, chopped

1 medium onion, thinly sliced

1 15-oz can chopped tomatoes

1 cup of chopped, roasted red pepper

1 tbsp balsamic vinegar

1 ½ cup reduced-fat ricotta

1 tbsp grated lemon rind

4 oz shredded, cooked (boiled) chicken

4 oz grated, reduced-fat cheese

1. In large pot of boiling water cook pasta 8 to 10 minutes until tender. Drain and set aside.

2. Meanwhile in large nonstick pan add zucchini, green pepper and onion over medium heat, stirring frequently until tender. Add canned tomatoes, red pepper and vinegar. Simmer 10 to 15 minutes until sauce thickens. Stir in pasta and set aside.

3. Preheat oven to 350°F, spray a 9 x 13 inch baking pan with cooking spray.

4. In a medium bowl, combine ricotta and lemon.

5. Arrange half of the pasta in prepared pan, spread ricotta mixture on top and sprinkle with chicken, top with remaining pasta mixture and sprinkle with grated cheese. Bake for 30 minutes until heated through and bubbly.

Nutrition Information Per Serving: 367 calories, 33g carbs, 31g protein, 6g fiber, 13g fat

Tuna Lentil Patties

SERVES 6

6 medium-sized potatoes, mashed

3 5-oz cans of tuna

2 cups of cooked lentils

1 chopped onion

1 chopped carrot

1 chopped red pepper, or green, or both

1 cup chopped parsley, or half a cup of dry parsley

¼ cup oregano, dry or fresh

½ cup lemon juice

2 egg whites

salt and pepper to taste

whole-wheat flour for dusting

paprika to taste

1. Mix all ingredients except flour and paprika together.

2. Roll in whole-wheat flour seasoned with paprika into any size balls you like. Dust work surface with whole-wheat flour seasoned with paprika. One spoonful at a time, roll the mixture over work surface into balls of your desired size.

3. Spray oil onto a flat baking sheet and bake at 300°F for 20 minutes, until golden brown. You can also fry the balls in a nonstick frying pan, lightly sprayed with oil.

Nutrition Information Per Serving: 283 calories, 49g carbs, 19g protein, 13g fiber, 1g fat

Low-Fat Cheese and Bacon Puffs

MAKES 12 PUFFS

2 cups plain whole-wheat flour

2 tsp baking powder

1 cup grated low-fat cheese

1 cup of diced turkey bacon, trimmed of all fat

1 cup skim milk

2 eggs

1. Preheat oven to 400°F.

2. Sift flour with baking powder, then stir in cheese and turkey bacon.

3. Mix milk and eggs together in separate bowl. Add to flour mixture, stirring until just combined; if too watery add extra flour.

4. Spoon into paper-lined muffin tin and bake at 400°F for 15 to 20 minutes.

Nutrition Information Per Serving: 140 calories, 17g carbs, 9g protein, 1g fiber, 4g fat

Porcupine Meat Ball

SERVES 6

26 oz 95% lean ground beef

½ cup uncooked brown rice

1 diced onion

1 tsp mixed herbs

1 tsp beef bouillon powder

1 cup evaporated milk

1 16-oz can of tomato soup

1 cup of water

Salt and pepper

1. Mix meat, rice, onion, seasonings and milk together.
2. Shape into little balls and brown in a nonstick pan.
3. Heat tomato soup and water to boiling point.
4. Drop meatballs into liquid, cover and simmer gently for 30 minutes.

Nutrition Information Per Serving: 278 calories, 16g carbs, 30g protein, 1g fiber, 10g fat

Pita Bread Pizza

SERVES 2

1 medium-sized pita bread	1 handful pineapple pieces
2 tsp tomato paste	1 handful sliced mushrooms
½ handful shredded ham	1 handful light shredded cheese
½ onion, diced	pinch of oregano
1 green pepper, diced	pinch of basil

1. Preheat oven to 350°F.
2. Prepare pita bread by spreading tomato paste evenly.
3. Sprinkle shredded ham, onion, green pepper, pineapple and mushrooms over the pita base. Cover with shredded cheese and add pinches of oregano and basil.
4. Bake pizza at 350°F for 15 to 20 minutes.

   The pita bread pizza ingredients are not limited to the above. Prepare your pizza toppings to your liking but make sure that the ingredients are healthy choices.

Nutrition Information Per Serving: 361 calories, 19g carbs, 28g protein, 3g fiber, 19g fat

Karen's Super Easy Sauce

SERVES 4

This is a sauce I love to make that is great over beef patties, chicken, pork, fish and mashed potatoes.

1 16-oz can crushed tomatoes

1 cube chicken bouillon

pinch of curry and pepper

Mix together in a medium saucepan and simmer gently for a few minutes until heated through, then serve over your meal.

Nutrition Information Per Serving: 36 calories, 8g carbs, 2g protein, 2g fiber, 0g fat

Low-Fat Macaroni and Cheese

SERVES 4

1 package uncooked whole-wheat elbow macaroni

½ tbsp flour

2 cups skim milk

1 ¼ cups reduced-fat cheddar cheese, grated

1 tsp mustard

freshly ground black pepper

1. Cook pasta according to the instructions on the package.

2. While pasta is cooking, place flour in a medium saucepan and gradually whisk in milk. Heat the milk and flour over medium heat and bring to a boil, stirring constantly to prevent lumps.

3. Reduce heat and allow to simmer until the milk begins to thicken. Stir in cheese and mustard, and continue to stir until cheese melts. Toss drained pasta and sauce in a large bowl. Add freshly ground black pepper and serve immediately.

Nutrition Information Per Serving: 257 calories, 38g carbs, 20g protein, 3g fiber, 4g fat

Grilled Chicken with Greek Salad

SERVES 4

2 tbsp low-fat yogurt

juice of 1 lemon

1 tbsp Greek seasoning

2 tbsp mint leaves, finely chopped

1 lb chicken tenderloins, tendons removed, trimmed

olive oil cooking spray

3 ½ oz baby spinach

3 ½ oz roasted pepper, sliced

1 cucumber, roughly chopped

1 ½ oz snow pea sprouts

2 oz low-fat feta cheese, crumbled

½ cup kalamata olives in brine

1. Mix yogurt, 2 teaspoons lemon juice, Greek seasoning and mint in a bowl. Add chicken and turn to coat. Cover and refrigerate for 20 minutes.

2. Preheat a barbecue grill on medium-low heat. Remove chicken from marinade and spray lightly with oil. Barbecue for 2 to 3 minutes each side or until just cooked through.

3. Meanwhile, place spinach, pepper, cucumber, sprouts, feta and olives in a bowl. Toss to combine. Divide salad among plates. Top with chicken. Drizzle with remaining lemon juice. Season with pepper. Serve.

Nutrition Information Per Serving: 216 calories, 9g carbs, 30g protein, 2g fiber, 7g fat

Chicken and Ricotta Cannelloni

SERVES 6

1 tbsp olive oil	good pinch nutmeg
1 small onion, finely chopped	4 fresh lasagne sheets
2 garlic cloves, crushed	24 oz jar Italian tomato sauce
14 oz ground chicken	½ cup grated cheese
10 oz low-fat ricotta	3 oz mixed salad greens, to serve

1. Preheat oven to 350°F. Heat olive oil in a nonstick frypan over medium heat. Add onion and garlic, cooking for 2 minutes until soft.

2. Add ground chicken. Cook until it changes color, breaking lumps with a wooden spoon.

3. Transfer to a bowl and allow to cool. Add ricotta and nutmeg and season with salt and pepper. Mix well.

4. Cut each lasagne sheet in half, forming two small rectangles. Place ⅓ cup of chicken mixture on one long side of the pasta, about 1 inch in from the edge. Roll up.

5. Spread half the tomato sauce evenly over the base of 4 individual or 1 large baking dish. Arrange cannelloni in dish. Spoon remaining sauce on top and sprinkle with cheese. Bake for 35 minutes until pasta is cooked. Serve with salad greens.

Nutrition Information Per Serving: 280 calories, 15g carbs, 24g protein, 3g fiber, 15g fat

Low-Fat Pasta Carbonara

SERVES 4

14 oz dried whole-wheat fettuccine or spaghetti

olive oil cooking spray

5 oz turkey bacon, thinly sliced

1 large brown onion, finely chopped

3 eggs

2 oz low-fat parmesan cheese, finely grated

2 tbsp flat-leaf parsley, chopped

salt and pepper to taste

1. Cook pasta in a large saucepan of boiling salted water, following package directions, until just tender.

2. Meanwhile, lightly spray a frying pan with oil. Heat over medium heat. Add bacon and onion. Cook, stirring, for 3 to 4 minutes, or until golden.

3. Drain pasta and return immediately to hot saucepan. Whisk eggs in a bowl with a fork. Add to hot pasta. Stir quickly to coat pasta.

4. Add bacon mixture, parmesan, parsley and salt and pepper to pasta. Toss over low heat for 1 to 2 minutes, or until heated through. Serve immediately.

Nutrition Information Per Serving: 336 calories, 33g carbs, 21g protein, 5g fiber, 15g fat

Mediterranean Meat Loaf

SERVES 4

½ cup brown rice

1 small red onion, grated

12 oz 95% lean ground beef

1 carrot, peeled, grated

2 oz low-fat feta cheese, crumbled

2 tbsp tomato sauce

1 tbsp Worcestershire sauce

1 egg, lightly beaten

2 tbsp basil leaves, shredded (or 2 tsp dried basil)

1 zucchini, thinly sliced

13 oz cherry tomatoes

1 garlic clove, crushed

olive oil cooking spray

1. Cook rice following absorption method on packet. Set aside to cool.

2. Preheat oven to 400°F. Grease base and sides of a 3-inch-deep, 9 x 5 inch loaf pan. Line with baking paper, allowing a 1-inch overhang at both long ends.

3. Combine rice, onion, ground beef, carrot, feta, sauces, egg and basil in a bowl. Mix well. Press into prepared pan.

4. Place zucchini, tomatoes and garlic in a bowl. Spray with oil. Toss to combine. Spoon over meat loaf. Bake for 60 to 80 minutes or until meat loaf is firm. Let stand for 10 minutes. Slice and serve.

Nutrition Information Per Serving: 212 calories, 14g carbs, 22g protein, 2g fiber, 7g fat

Sun-Dried Tomato and Spinach Pie

SERVES 8

¼ cup olive oil

3 brown onions, halved, finely chopped

1 leek, pale section only, washed, dried, thinly sliced

1 bunch spinach, white stems removed, washed with water clinging to leaves

9 oz low-fat ricotta

½ cup finely grated low-fat parmesan

5 oz sun-dried tomatoes, soaked in warm water for 2 hours

2 eggs, lightly whisked

salt and freshly ground black pepper

16 sheets phyllo pastry

4 oz reduced-fat dairy spread, melted

1. Preheat oven to 350°F. Brush a 9 x 13 inch pan with oil to lightly grease.

2. Heat oil in a frying pan over medium heat. Add onion and leek. Cook, stirring, for 5 minutes or until onion softens.

3. Place spinach in a saucepan over low heat. Cook, covered, for 2 minutes or until wilted. Remove from heat and set aside for 5 minutes to cool. Squeeze out any excess liquid. Finely chop.

4. Combine onion mixture, spinach, ricotta, parmesan, tomatoes and egg in a bowl, and season with salt and pepper.

5. Place phyllo on a clean surface. Cover with a dry tea towel, then a damp tea towel (this will prevent it from drying out). Brush 1 phyllo sheet with melted dairy spread. Top with another sheet and brush that with dairy spread. Continue layering with 6 more sheets to make a stack. Repeat with remaining phyllo and spread to make a second stack.

(continued)

6. Line prepared pan with 1 phyllo stack, allowing it to overhang. Spread with onion mixture. Top with remaining phyllo stack and gently scrunch edges together to enclose filling. Bake in preheated oven for 45 minutes or until golden. Remove from oven. Set aside for 5 minutes to cool slightly. Cut into 8 squares to serve.

Nutrition Information Per Serving: 346 calories, 38g carbs, 14g protein, 4g fiber, 17g fat

Low-Fat Beef "Olives"

SERVES 8

1 ½ cups fresh whole-wheat bread crumbs

½ cup sun-dried tomatoes, soaked in warm water for 2 hours, roughly chopped

½ cup grated low-fat parmesan cheese

¼ cup basil leaves, finely shredded (or 4 tsp dried basil)

2 tbsp toasted pine nuts

1 egg, beaten

salt and pepper, to taste

4 thin (6 oz each) lean topside steaks

2 tbsp olive oil

2 cups beef stock

1. Combine bread crumbs, sun-dried tomato, low-fat parmesan, basil, pine nuts, egg and salt and pepper in a bowl.

2. Cut each steak in half, creating 2 thinner steaks. Place a piece of steak between 2 sheets plastic wrap. Using a meat mallet, pound until very thin. Spoon 2 tablespoonfuls bread mixture onto one end of steak. Fold in sides and roll up. Secure with toothpicks. Repeat with remaining steaks and bread mixture.

3. Heat oil in a large frying pan over medium-high heat. Cook the beef olives you just made in batches, for 2 to 3 minutes or until browned. Transfer to a plate.

4. Pour stock into the pan and bring to a boil. Return beef olives to pan. Reduce heat to medium-low. Simmer, turning occasionally, for 10 minutes or until cooked through. Transfer beef to a plate. Cover with foil.

5. Increase heat to high. Simmer sauce for 5 minutes or until thickened slightly. Remove toothpicks. Place beef olives on plates. Spoon sauce onto them and serve with steamed vegetables, if desired.

Nutrition Information Per Serving: 355 calories, 18g carbs, 32g protein, 2g fiber, 17g fat

---

DELICIOUS DESSERTS

Broiled Peaches with Ricotta

SERVES 4

---

4 just-ripe freestone peaches,
halved, pit removed

7 oz fresh low-fat ricotta cheese

pinch ground cinnamon

3 Sesame Snaps (or low-fat
cookies), crushed

1 tbsp honey, to serve

---

1. Preheat broiler on medium-high heat. Line a baking tray with nonstick baking paper. Place peaches, cut side up, on tray.

2. Place the ricotta, cinnamon and ¾ of the sesame snaps in a bowl. Stir until well combined. Spoon mixture into peach cavities. Sprinkle remaining Sesame Snaps over the top. Broil peaches for 4 to 5 minutes or until Sesame Snaps melt.

3. Drizzle honey over peaches and serve.

Nutrition Information Per Serving: 244 calories, 40g carbs, 8g protein,
3g fiber, 7g fat

Cherry & Berry Slushies

SERVES 4

¾ cup water

⅓ cup caster (superfine) sugar

2 tbsp fresh lemon juice

10 oz pitted fresh or thawed frozen cherries

9 oz strawberries, washed, hulled

1. Combine the water, sugar and lemon juice in a small saucepan and stir over low heat for 1 minute or until the sugar dissolves (see microwave tip).

2. Place the sugar mixture, cherries and strawberries in the bowl of a food processor or blender and process until smooth. Pour the mixture into a shallow freezer-proof container and freeze for 3 to 4 hours or until almost frozen.

3. Break the mixture up with a spoon and place in the bowl of a food processor and process until smooth. Pour into four 1-cup plastic, freezer-proof cups. Cover with foil and place in the freezer overnight.

Microwave Tip: *Place the water, sugar and lemon juice in a 2-cup heatproof, microwave-safe jug or bowl. Cook on high for 1 minute, stirring occasionally, until sugar dissolves.*

Nutrition Information Per Serving: 124 calories, 32g carbs, 1g protein, 3g fiber, 0g fat

Grilled Fruit Skewers

SERVES 4

1 small, ripe mango

¼ small pineapple, peeled, sliced into inch-thick wedges

5 oz strawberries, hulled, halved

1 banana, cut into inch-thick slices

¼ cup passion-fruit pulp (optional, see tip)

5 oz low-fat strawberry yogurt

1. Preheat grill on medium-high heat. Slice 2 cheeks* from mango. Cut each cheek into 6 cubes. Remove skin.

2. Thread mango, pineapple, strawberries and banana alternately onto skewers. Line barbecue plate with baking paper (see tip). Barbecue skewers, turning often, for 3 to 4 minutes or until warmed through.

3. Place 1 skewer on each plate. Drizzle with passion-fruit pulp. Serve warm with yogurt.

Tip: *You will need 4 presoaked bamboo skewers. Baking paper will prevent fruit from sticking to barbecue plate and burning. You will need 2 passion fruit for ¼ cup pulp.*

Nutrition Information Per Serving: 147 calories, 36g carbs, 3g protein, 5g fiber, 1g fat

* Cheek = ½ mango sliced lengthwise off pit.

Custard Apples

SERVES 4

4 small Granny Smith apples	¼ cup apple juice
1 ½ tbsp minced fruit (mixed dried fruit such as raisins or sultanas)	¼ cup mango juice
	½ cup low-fat vanilla yogurt

1. Preheat oven to 350°F. Using an apple corer, core apples. Slice around the middle of each apple to prevent bursting during cooking (see tip).

2. Place apples in a ceramic baking dish. Spoon minced fruit into apple centers. Pour juice over the apples. Bake for 25 to 30 minutes or until apples are just tender, basting every 10 minutes with juice.

3. Divide apples between serving plates. Spoon juice over them and serve with yogurt.

Tip: *Baking apples: To prevent apples exploding during baking, use a sharp knife to cut a ¼-inch-deep circle around the top, middle and base of each apple. This also allows heat to penetrate the fruit, reducing the cooking time.*

Nutrition Information Per Serving: 139 calories, 34g carbs, 2g protein, 4g fiber, 1g fat

Berry Jell-O

SERVES 4

1 package low-calorie raspberry Jell-O

1 cup boiling water

9 oz strawberries, hulled, sliced

5 oz blueberries

1 ½ cups prepared, low-fat vanilla pudding

1. Place Jell-O in a jug. Add boiling water and stir until completely dissolved. Stir in 1 cup cold water.

2. Pour Jell-O into four 1-cup-capacity glasses. Spoon half the strawberries and blueberries into Jell-O. Cover and refrigerate for at least 4 hours or until set.

3. Top Jell-O with remaining strawberries and blueberries and pudding. Serve.

Nutrition Information Per Serving: 116 calories, 25g carbs, 2g protein, 2g fiber, 0g fat

Yummy Baked Apples

SERVES 1 APPLE PER PERSON

1 jar fat-free minced fruit (mixed dried fruit, such as raisins, sultanas)

cored apples (peel the skin only if you don't like the apple skin, otherwise leave)

cinnamon, nutmeg, allspice to dust

1. Preheat oven to 400°F.

2. Spoon or pipe the minced fruit into the holes of the apples.

3. Place into a deep dish and fill the dish ¼ full of water.

4. Sprinkle with cinnamon, nutmeg and allspice and cover with waxed paper.

5. Bake in preheated oven for 20 minutes.

6. Test with a skewer or knife—if it goes in easily, they're ready. Be sure not to cook them too long or they'll become too soft.

7. Serve with fat-free pudding or yogurt and have a yummy, guilt-free warm winter dessert!

Nutrition Information Per Serving: 177 calories, 42g carbs, 4g protein, 3g fiber, 0g fat

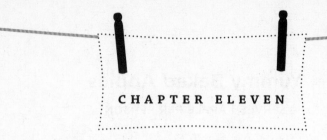

CHAPTER ELEVEN

All of Your Diet Questions Answered

ONE OF THE THINGS I HAVE LEARNED SINCE LOSING WEIGHT IS that the questions I was asking through my journey are the same questions every dieter seems to have. Regardless of whether it's 20 or 200 pounds you need to lose, the issues that plague us are all the same. So here is a list of the most common questions I get asked and my answers. These aren't textbook theories—they are tried-and-tested practical solutions to everyday questions that worked for me. I hope they will be useful to you, too!

I find it really difficult to drink plain water. What can I have instead?

There are great low-sugar mixes available that have the same flavor as the full-sugar blends. Or buy freshly squeezed grapefruit and orange juices from the supermarket. But nothing beats water, so aim for at least six to eight glasses every day. Try squeezing a little fresh lemon, grapefruit or orange juice into your water. This gives it a nice lift and will help you adjust quickly to drinking water.

What do I do when my weight reaches a plateau and I'm not losing anymore?

You must look at your diet and exercise routine, and deduct food or add action. For example, if you usually have two pieces of bread in a sandwich for lunch, make an open-faced sandwich with the same filling, using a large rice cake instead of bread. Or add a little to your walk or other exercise each day. Make the effort to exercise for an extra five or ten minutes—as much as you can do.

I always reached a plateau every three months or so when, for about two weeks, I would stop losing weight. That's when I knew I had to play around with my diet and make a few adjustments. A lot of people give up their diet during the plateau stage. It's a very dangerous time, and you can lose your motivation quite quickly if you think you are not losing weight. But it's really just a simple case of fine-tuning your weight-loss plan, and you'll find that in no time the pounds will start to come off again.

How do I beat cravings?

To beat cravings, stay positive and focus on your goals and dreams. Cravings can be hard to resist but, remember, it's just your mind playing tricks on you, not your tummy. I constantly craved sweet food—that's why I dipped my finger in sugar and enjoyed that to beat the craving. But tell yourself, *it's my mind, not my tummy.* You have to fight the cravings; don't let them beat you. Ask yourself, *am I really hungry?* Nine times out of ten you won't be—it's all in your mind.

When can I eat carbohydrates?

You've all heard of, and probably tried, low-carb, or carb-free diets, right? Maybe these diets work for some, but I'm guessing if you're reading my book, the no-carb/low-carb fad hasn't worked for you. I ate carbohydrates every day while I was dieting, I ate them whenever I wanted. I didn't restrict myself to set periods of the day when I could or could not eat carbohydrates. With two little children to cook for I couldn't cook meals for them and meals for me—it wasn't practical. But it's all about moderation, so I just cut my portions down. If we had pasta or mashed potatoes for dinner, I ate them—I just ate smaller portions of them than I used to.

How do I know what is healthy when I go shopping for food?

I always look for low-fat or fat-free products. Just about every food has a low-fat version, so look out for them and read the labels carefully. For example, cheeses. I compared them all and bought the lowest-fat version I could find.

The first few shopping trips will take you longer than normal because you need to consider the food you're buying, but once you get the hang of it, it will take no time at all. Look for alternatives; don't just accept what is in front of you on the shelf. Also be careful to check the sugar content, because some foods may well be fat-free or low in fat, but have a high sugar content. Use your common sense and buy as much fresh food as you can. But I have to stress again, just because it's fat-free, this doesn't mean you can eat twice as much!

Can I drink any milk other than fat-free milk?

Yes, absolutely. There are lots of different low-fat milks available, so take your pick. It took me a while to find one I liked. A little of it is trial and error, depending on your or your family's tastes. When I first began, fat-free milk tasted like water to me, but I got used to it very quickly.

How do I stay motivated?

Believe in yourself. You have to take control of your life and tell yourself *I deserve a better life. I deserve to lose my weight.* Staying motivated is hard; you really have to concentrate on your goal and visualize yourself in the future. Get a picture in your mind of how you'd like to look in six months' time and use that to work toward your goal. Constantly remind yourself that you can achieve anything and you will. And set smaller goals to achieve step-by-step along the way. As you achieve them, you'll feel a great sense of satisfaction and this will drive you to achieve the next goal.

Why do I eat more when I'm feeling depressed?

When you are depressed, food seems to be a comfort, especially when you are depressed about your weight. People eat for comfort. We eat when we're bored, when we're sad. We eat if we're lonely. But we often don't realize that we are eating for these reasons rather than because we are hungry. You must gain control of the food—I've said this many times throughout the book and I honestly can't repeat it enough. Don't let the food control you.

You have to overcome depression to begin losing weight. It's harsh but it's true. Address the issues in your life that are making you depressed and sort through them; then as you gain control of your life, the depression will lift and you will no longer turn to food for comfort.

People always say to me, "But you're always happy, you're never depressed," but I do have my down days like everybody else. When I was at my highest weight, although I was always smiling and happy on the outside, I was at rock bottom on the inside.

These days, I have control over my life, and I won't eat to feel better about an issue. I sort out the issue that is preying on my mind, so it's not in the equation anymore. I have control, and you must take control, too.

Do I have to eat breakfast?

Absolutely! Having breakfast is so important, it gets you going and gives you the energy you need for the day. It's like going to the gas station and filling your car up—it gets your metabolism going and gets you on the move. You must make sure that you get that engine started in the morning so there's no stopping you for the rest of the day.

Do I have to eat three meals a day?

Yes. As I mentioned above, you must have breakfast to kick-start the day, and lunch and dinner are equally as important. Do not starve yourself. If you don't eat three meals a day you will spend your day picking at food and that's dangerous. When you pick you have no control over the amount you're eating. I want you to enjoy your food, too, not feel like you're grabbing something on the run.

When you're picking at food you don't care what you eat, either. You're more inclined to just go to the cupboard and grab whatever is there rather than think about what you are eating. Take the time to prepare food, sit down and enjoy it. Enjoy your evening dinner with your family or your partner—it's precious time to catch up with the people you love or to take some time to yourself to reflect on the day. If you're at work, prepare your lunch before you go. Take a healthy sandwich and some fruit or pack a salad.

A lot of people tell me they prefer to have six small meals through the day rather than eating large meals because they get hungry in between. With my seven-day diet plan I include a lot of snacks in between meals. Six small meals a day is fine, as long as the food you eat is healthy, not junk food that you grab because it's convenient.

Why do I eat more when I have my period?

Sorry, girls, you'll hate me for saying this, but I honestly believe women use their periods as an excuse to binge every month, and it's not necessary. It's all in our minds. It's a little bit like pregnancy—we use it as an excuse to eat much more than we normally would and eat foods that we normally wouldn't. "I'm eating for two" sound familiar? There's no doubt that we do become more tired when we have our period and we do feel a little more run-down, but that doesn't mean we can attack the fridge with gusto.

You don't overcome tiredness by eating more. I suggest instead that you have a nap in the afternoon or have a few extra minutes in bed in the morning, but don't use your period as an excuse to plow through chocolate bars and candies. No, no, no.

Is your diet recommended by doctors?

This is a diet that is based on common sense and, although it hasn't undergone years of medical research, my doctor gave me the thumbs-up and encouraged me to follow this plan. I developed it to help me lose my weight, and it worked. And it works for other people, too. There are no radical steps you have to take, no starvation and no bizarre eating rituals. It's all just common sense.

Having said that, I strongly suggest that everyone who wants to begin any diet, not just mine, see their doctor first. I strongly encourage you to take this plan to your doctor and talk it through. I found it very helpful to have my doctor's support. He weighed me and checked my progress, and my regular appointments with him were very motivating for me.

Not everybody sticks rigidly to my eating plan—some people simply don't like the foods I eat—so I encourage you to exchange the foods I suggest with other low-fat foods that you enjoy. Although you won't find pages and pages of medical research on the Clothesline Diet you will find that it is a very practical, easy-to-follow, commonsense plan that works!

Why is it that I walk for an hour a day and I eat healthy food, but I don't seem to lose weight?

It's simply because your body is used to the same routine. I suggest you vary your routine, introducing a new element (gradually, of course) such as walking a little bit faster for part of the time. Instead of walking comfortably along for thirty minutes, try power walking for fifteen minutes to change it up. You will soon begin to see the pounds drop.

Keep an eye on your diet, too; when you reach a plateau, you may need to modify what you are eating. If you follow my diet to the letter and the pounds don't seem to be budging, don't get turned off because there is a good chance you will be losing inches instead of pounds. Many of the people I speak to have found that after two or three weeks the weight loss will begin to be noticeable on the scales, too. But you must also allow your body time to adjust and react to the exercise, water and healthy food. Don't be disheartened if you aren't seeing instant results. Effective weight loss takes time. After all, it's taken time to accumulate all of the pounds. The loss will be gradual and consistent but the pounds will stay off! Weight loss isn't supposed to happen overnight.

Is any fruit or vegetable bad to eat?

My answer is no. Eat as much fruit and as many vegetables as you can, but remember that some fruits have more sugar than others, so do limit those. Fruits like bananas, grapes and mangoes can be high in natural sugar. For that reason I only have two bananas a week, and vegetables such as potatoes and squash can be high in carbohydrates, too, so keep an eye on your intake. I'd still rather you reach for grapes or a mango than a slab of chocolate, though!

Does it make a difference what time I exercise during the day?

No, as long as you exercise for twenty minutes to half an hour each day. But you should have something before you exercise, even if it's only a cup of tea. Don't wake up with an empty stomach and go straight out for a walk, or you may get dizzy or feel faint. You need a little bit of fuel to get the engine going!

When I get down to my goal weight will I end up with excess skin?

That's a very hard question to answer because everybody is different. When I lost my weight I ended up with a lot of excess skin, especially around my tummy and the back of my arms, and I found that very depressing. I'd worked so hard and I'd lost all of this weight, and yet I had this flap of skin sitting on my belly. So on the advice of my doctor I had it removed.

I had excess skin because I had been so big all of my life, there was virtually no elasticity left in my skin. I started putting on weight when I was four years old, so my skin was really stretched and simply wouldn't go back into shape. But I know of many women who have lost a lot of weight, some well over 120 or 130 pounds, and have had no excess skin at all. Their skin had retained elasticity and they haven't had a problem. It really does depend on you. But don't let the thought of excess skin deter you from losing your weight!

Do I have to follow your plan to the letter?

No, it is just a guide, a basic health plan that you can work with. There are a lot of different products on the supermarket shelf that you can choose from. Mix and match and use the plan as a learning tool to eat, shop and live a healthy life.

Do you recommend set mealtimes?

No, I never had specific mealtimes. I ate breakfast when I got up, lunch when I wanted to, but usually between noon and two, and dinner when I could manage to get Jason and the kids in one room at the same time! Some people work shifts or just work odd hours, so you can't be rigid about these things. I do recommend having your evening meal early, though, so you can do some sort of activity afterward: go for a walk, to the gym or to the park. That way, you are not sitting on your bottom for the whole night! Don't sit watching TV on a full stomach. It'll only turn to fat.

Can I do the Clothesline Diet if I don't have a clothesline?

Yes! Can you believe people ask this question? And yet I hear it all the time: "I can't do your diet. I don't have a clothesline." It's the laziest excuse I've ever heard!

My clothesline was the tool I used to help get me started because I was too embarrassed to walk out on the street, and I really couldn't manage to walk any farther than a few steps at first. I know people who walk up and down hallways in their houses, do water aerobics or walk laps at a nearby track. One lady lives in the Outback and lost her weight by walking along the dirt track through the desert to her mailbox each day! Some people who have two-story homes walk up and down the stairs. It's really about finding the exercise you are happy with and enjoy doing. As I've said before, whether that's riding a bike, going for a jog or walking around the clothesline, it doesn't matter. This is just a guide to get you on your way. And remember, if I can do it, anyone can!

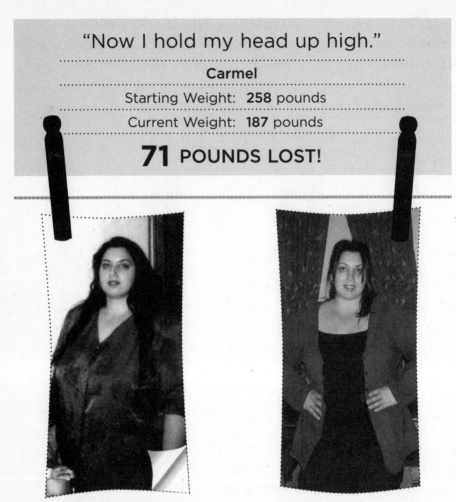

"Now I hold my head up high."

Carmel

Starting Weight: **258** pounds

Current Weight: **187** pounds

71 POUNDS LOST!

I heard Karen speak in a radio interview a few years ago and I was instantly inspired. My weight really was out of control and I was so unhappy. I hated myself and I hated how I was treating my husband and children. I was always grumpy, always yelling and angry. I was taking my frustration out on them, and I really didn't like the person I'd become. I felt like I was at war with them and the world.

But what really prompted me to lose weight was when my mum had her first heart scare at the age of thirty-nine. Like Mum, I was feeling a few unusual things in my chest and I automatically thought I was going down the same road. It was really scary and it probably took the thought that I was following in Mum's footsteps to shake me into reality.

Karen is amazing. She's a wonderful person and she made me see that we are all special no matter what size we are. Karen gave me a reason to live and find myself.

She gave me the tools I needed to start my road to health. After losing my weight, I was able to play and laugh again with my family. I no longer look down or away when people are talking to me, and I feel full of confidence. Now I hold my head up high and live every day. I make the most of life with my family and I love the world again.

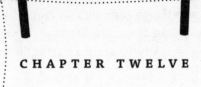

CHAPTER TWELVE

Tried and True:

Foolproof Tips and Helpful Hints for Success

FOR ME, LOSING SO MUCH WEIGHT SEEMED TO PHYSICALLY LIFT a darkness, a fog, that had surrounded me for as long as I could remember. And the key to my success was as much about new ways of thinking as it was physical changes. I'm still learning every day of my life, and I want to share some of my thoughts and some advice that has been helpful to my support group and to other Clothesline Dieters in their journeys from obesity.

These are tried-and-true tips. I used them while I was losing my weight and I still live by them today. You will find your own helpful tricks as you go along your journey, too. Write them down so that when you're having a bad day you can have a quick read over your tips to motivate yourself and get back on the right track.

- Take each day as it comes and address each problem as it arises; don't let problems accumulate until you feel you can't cope with them. Deal with the problem and move on with your life. The longer a problem lingers the greater it will become, so nip it in the bud and get it out of the way.

- Stress causes depression and, thanks to emotional eating, depression causes weight gain. If you are feeling particularly stressed, take a little time for yourself, but don't head to the pantry! Sit down for five minutes and do your nails, phone a friend and have coffee or see a movie. Go for a long walk or just find a quiet place at home and sit on the floor for five minutes while you take some long deep breaths. The pantry should be the last place on your list of places to head because it will only add to your stress. Food does not provide emotional comfort.

- Live life to the fullest. Enjoy every minute of every day—life is too short not to! I can't say this enough. Life shouldn't be a chore—smile and enjoy it. And if you're not enjoying your life, take time to work out why. Pour a cup of tea, sit down and have a think. Make a list of all of the things you do not like about your life and why, then work out ways you can turn the negatives into positives. Life will soon seem much more enjoyable.

Live life to the fullest. Enjoy every minute of every day—life is too short not to!

- Make time for those moments that count: helping the kids with their homework, playing games or having a coffee with friends.

- Before you begin, tell yourself over and over again "I believe in me." Fight for your goals—we can all achieve what we want to in life if we only believe in ourselves. If you have the faith within, you can achieve your dreams.

If you have the faith within, you can achieve your dreams.

- Make time for more family activities: playing in the park, kicking a football, swimming, going to the beach. The bond between you and your family will grow, and you'll feel healthier and happier.

- Ignore smart remarks that others might make when they find out you are trying to lose weight. People are always quick to judge and can be very negative. I often heard people saying "She'll never do it," "She's always been fat," "Here she goes again." Those attitudes can be hurtful, but instead of letting them get you down, use them as motivation! Smile inside in anticipation of the looks on their faces when you achieve your goal. Use others' cynicism to drive you toward your goal—prove the doubters wrong!

Stay focused at all times on achieving your goal. Prove the doubters wrong.

- When losing your weight, stay focused at all times on achieving your goal. I've seen many instances where people lose focus halfway to their goal weight because everybody begins to compliment them and they think they can stop working at it. Inevitably the weight begins to creep back up and, more often than not, they end up right back where they started. Stay focused and don't let the compliments get in the way of your ultimate goal.

- Instead of eating chocolate, eat 99 percent fat-free licorice, or gummy worms. If you are desperate for chocolate and feel you can't possibly exist without it, eat chocolate-coated licorice bites—but only a few at a time. Don't make a habit of it, rather use them just to satisfy the craving. There are many low-fat candies on the market and I always buy fat-free licorice and gummy worms. The kids like them, too.

  There is no such thing as "I can't."

- When you are walking, take a bottle of water with you, and make it your goal to come home with the bottle empty. As your walking progresses, challenge yourself to drink more water.

- Make your walk a part of your everyday routine. Just as you get out of bed, have a shower and make a cup of coffee each day, your walk should be a routine thing.

- Leave a full bowl of fruit salad in the fridge for whenever you may get hungry, and snack on it regularly. Prepare the fruit salad when you are not hungry. That way, when the munchies hit, the fruit is ready to go and you're not tempted to grab something quickly off the shelf.

- When you go to restaurants, look at the menu and take time to really look for healthy foods before you order. Don't be afraid to ask the chef to cook the meal in a different way or to cook a meal that may not be on the menu. Most restaurants are accommodating, especially if you explain you are trying to lose weight.

- Have two to three glasses of water before your lunch and dinner. It will make you feel full before you've even begun to eat.

- If it's cold and raining outside and you just don't feel like heading out for a walk, remember you do have a raincoat, you do have an umbrella—there is no excuse! There is no such thing as "I can't."

- If you have children, take them with you on your walk. It's much more fun than walking on your own and you'll probably burn up more fat. Children should never be an excuse for not exercising—instead they should be a great resource for burning calories!

- Don't let food control you. You have to learn to control it.

- The simplest way to begin a successful diet is not to cut everything out. Just replace bad food with good. I replaced fatty foods with low-fat versions of the same meals and I never felt like I was missing out on anything!

- Discuss your diet plans with your doctor and have a full health check before you begin. My doctor was a great help to me and a huge support. I made regular appointments to check my progress and each time I could see big improvements in my blood pressure and general health. The weeks when I hadn't lost much weight, it was still a real bonus to hear that my blood pressure was going down or that the swelling in my legs and feet was decreasing. With each visit I could see I was achieving my goal!

> *Don't let food control you. You have to learn to control it.*

> *Reward yourself with a treat when you achieve small goals.*

- Cut out soft drinks completely; they're a big no-no. With each meal have water or fruit juice, not soft drinks! If you think you can't do it, just picture yourself drinking a cup of sugar—because that's what you're doing!

- Reward yourself with a treat when you achieve small goals. For every five pounds I lost I allowed myself a little piece of chocolate—not the whole box, though! Enjoy, but don't overindulge.

- If you just have to have something sweet, dip the tip of your little finger in the sugar bowl and lick it. I know it probably sounds weird, but it really worked for me. That tiny amount will satisfy your craving. Don't dip your whole finger in, though—just the tip!

- Set little goals for yourself along the way and achieve them step-by-step. Buy a blouse you love that is one to two sizes smaller than your current size and work really hard to make it fit. When you've achieved your goal, your reward is a lovely new top that you've been longing to wear.

Set little goals for yourself along the way and achieve them step-by-step.

- And last, just because the food you are eating is much healthier, that doesn't mean you can eat twice as much. Your portions must remain small for each meal. Buy yourself a salad plate or a soup bowl—don't pile it high—and eat every meal from it.

One Last Word
Believing Is a Gift of Life

. . . .

I HOPE THIS BOOK INVIGORATES YOUR SPIRIT, TOUCHES YOUR soul and helps you find yourself. If you are walking down the road that I walked, hold your head up and look to the future. Follow in my footsteps and you will begin to see a new life for yourself. Life is beautiful and everybody deserves the chance to see how beautiful their world can be.

If there is one overwhelming truth I have learned from my journey, it is this: believing is a gift of life. The biggest gift you can give yourself in life is to believe in yourself because if you do, you can achieve anything.

Today I have new goals, and I'm going to work my hardest to achieve them.

My greatest ambition, though, is to help people who live as I once did. I want them to see and share the happiness I have experienced. Because if I can do it, anyone can.

Your Clothesline Diet Journal

CONGRATULATIONS ON TAKING THE FIRST STEP TO YOUR NEW LIFE!

When I started my diet, I weighed in at 283 pounds. I looked at that number on the scale and knew that I had a long way to go. But step by step, the pounds came off, along with the inches. And if I could do it, anyone can. Just like Rosetta, Laura, Lina, Aaron and the thousands of other Clothesline success stories, you have a success story in you just waiting to be told. It doesn't matter what you weigh now, so long as you follow the simple Clothesline Diet guidelines and stay motivated, the pounds will start to come off in no time!

Success doesn't happen overnight, and it helps to take an honest look at where you are and where you want to be, and to record all of your diet milestones along the way. This journal includes space to visualize your new life, write positive statements, set goals and track your progress. These are pages you can turn to again and again for inspiration. And someday you'll look back on these pages and think about how far you've come. Think of this as writing your own success story—and on the last page of this journal, that's exactly what you'll do. So let's make like a kangaroo and hop to it!

Visualize Your New Life

The day after the Mother's Day dance, before I cleaned out my pantry and stocked it with Clothesline Diet foods, I visualized how I wanted my new life to be. I imagined myself playing with my boys without getting tired, dancing with my husband with my head held high and wearing beautiful new clothes one day. Visualizing all of the amazing things I could do once I lost the weight really motivated me to change my life and take that first step.

You are about to start an incredible journey to a whole new you—how do you envision your new life? Once you lose the weight for good, what will you be able to do? Write it all down here and return to this journal page often to stay motivated and remind yourself of all you have to look forward to in your new life.

Believe in Yourself

The first step to your new life is believing in yourself. You *can* do this. Sure, you've tried other diets—so have I. But this diet really works. You just have to have faith in yourself that you will succeed and, first and foremost, remember all of the reasons that you deserve a better life.

Why I deserve a better life:

....

....

....

Stop the Negativity

We all have that little negative voice in our heads telling us that we aren't good enough. Just as I did, take your negative thoughts and turn them around.

Negative thought:

....

....

New positive thought:

....

....

Negative thought:

....

....

New positive thought:

....

....

Negative thought:

....

....

New positive thought:

....

....

Your Positive Statement

Every night before I went to bed, I'd stand in front of the mirror and look myself in the eye and say, "I deserve a better life. I want a better life. I can do this. Karen, you can do this." Eventually I started believing it myself. Create your own positive statement and repeat it every night as a reminder that you deserve to lose weight and that you can succeed:

....

....

....

....

....

Build Your Support Network

Having a support network makes dieting so much easier—and successful. I never would have achieved all that I did without Jason to support me. And our Clothesline Diet support group helps all of us stay motivated to lose the weight and keep it off. Whether you choose to start your own support group or prefer to have one person to lean on, take a minute to record your Clothesline Diet support network.

Name	Phone Number	E-mail Address

Before the Clothesline Diet

Every journey has a starting point. When I weighed nearly 300 pounds, it was hard to imagine that I'd ever weigh 155 pounds—but I do! And I'm so thankful that I kept track of every step of the journey, because knowing the milestones reminds me of how far I've really come. Time to start writing your own:

Date: On _____ ,
I am taking the very first step to change my life.

Starting Weight: _____

Goal Weight: _____

Before Photo:

Have Your (Low-Fat) Cake and Eat It, Too

The wonderful thing about the Clothesline Diet is that anyone can do it. You don't need any fancy food or equipment—all you have to do is follow the simple Clothesline rules and get moving. We all know that the more you deprive yourself, the more you crave something. So here's space for you to figure out how you'll replace the bad foods with good alternatives.

I will replace my favorite unhealthy foods for these healthier alternatives:

Unhealthy Food	Healthy Alternative

Step to It

Exercise is an important part of the Clothesline Diet, and once you get into the habit, it can be one of the most enjoyable parts of losing weight. I suggest exercising at least twenty minutes a day, five days a week. Don't worry if that seems like too much to start—remember, I could barely walk around my clothesline when I started!

You can always start with five minutes a day, and work your way up. Maybe twenty minutes doesn't seem like enough for you. You may prefer to exercise thirty minutes, or even forty-five. The key is figuring out what exercise you enjoy and then setting your goal.

Exercises and Activities I Enjoy:

....

....

....

....

My Exercise Goals

I want to exercise
_____ minutes a day, _____ times a week.

Right now, I can exercise
_____ minutes a day, _____ times a week.

To reach my goal, I will increase my exercise by
_____ minutes every day for _____ weeks.

Date I started:

Date I reached my goal:

Setting Small Goals

While I always had a goal weight in mind, it helped me to set small goals along the way. Whether it was lowering my blood pressure, getting into a new dress for my cousin's wedding or preparing for the new year, these goals gave me something to work for and small accomplishments to celebrate along the way.

Here is space to set your own goals:

My Goal	By Date/Event

Tracking Your Progress

Remember that it's never a good idea to weigh yourself once a day. Instead, I recommend weighing yourself once a week. Keeping track of how much you lose will help you stay motivated—it's encouraging to see those numbers go down!

week	1	2	3	4	5	6	7	8
weight								

Did you gain weight during the two-week maintaining period?

If so, what can you do differently next time?

Your Clothesline Diet Success Story

Congratulations on all of your hard work! Here is space for you to reflect on how far you've come—write your own success story.

My Success Story

Starting Weight: _____ pounds

Current Weight: _____ pounds

_____ **POUNDS LOST!**

After Photo:

My Story:

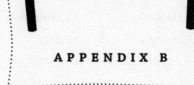

Metric Conversions

Converting to Metrics

VOLUME MEASUREMENT CONVERSIONS

U.S.	Metric
¼ teaspoon	1.25ml
½ teaspoon	2.5ml
¾ teaspoon	3.75ml
1 teaspoon	5ml
1 tablespoon	15ml
¼ cup	60ml
½ cup	120ml
¾ cup	180ml
1 cup	240ml

WEIGHT CONVERSIONS MEASUREMENT

U.S.	Metric
1 ounce	28g
8 ounces	230g
16 ounces (1 pound)	450g

COOKING TEMPERATURE CONVERSIONS

Celsius/Centigrade	0°C and 100°C are placed at the melting and boiling points of water respectively and are standard to the metric system.
Fahrenheit	Fahrenheit established 0°F as the stabilized temperature when equal amounts of ice, water and salt are mixed.

To convert temperatures in Fahrenheit to Celsius, use this formula: (°F–32) x 0.5555 = °C

So, for example, a recipe calls for the oven to be heated to 350°F and you want to know that temperature in Celsius, use this calculation: (350–32) x 0.5555 = 176.66°C

INDEX

C